REDUCING
CANCER MORTALITY
A Geographical Perspective

To Ken Stott

Teacher, Geographer and Friend

REDUCING CANCER MORTALITY
A Geographical Perspective

HAROLD D. FOSTER

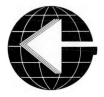

Western Geographical Series Volume 23

Department of Geography, University of Victoria
Victoria, British Columbia
Canada

1986 University of Victoria

Western Geographical Series, Volume 23

editorial address

Harold D. Foster, Ph.D.
Department of Geography
University of Victoria
Victoria, British Columbia
Canada

Publication of the Western Geographical Series has been gener-
ously supported by the Leon and Thea Koerner Foundation, the
Social Science Federation of Canada, the National Centre for
Atmospheric Research, the International Geographical Union Con-
gress, the University of Victoria and the Natural Sciences and
Engineering Research Council of Canada.

Foster, Harold D., 1943-
    REDUCING CANCER MORTALITY
(Western geographical series; ISSN 0315-2022; v. 23)
Bibliography: p.
ISBN 0-919838-13-8
1. Cancer - United States - Mortality. 2. Carcinogenesis. 3. Cancer
- Prevention. I. University of Victoria (B.C.), Dept. of Geography.
II. Title. III. Series.
RC276.F68 1986   614.5'999'0973   C86-091053-9

ACKNOWLEDGEMENTS

The author wishes to dedicate this book to Ken Stott, who as a senior master at the Hull Grammar School, first introduced him to the enormous potential of Geography. In addition, he would like to pay tribute to the countless millions who, over the centuries, have lost their lives to cancer. Hopefully, the hypotheses developed in this volume may assist in reducing the worldwide suffering, traditionally associated with this group of illnesses.

Many people have assisted the author in the collection of the data used in this study. These have included, for example, various members of the Department of Geography, University of Victoria, who have loaned literature or provided other aid. In particular, thanks is given to Dr. David Chuen-yan Lai for a map of the Geology of the People's Republic of China; Dr. Michael Edgell for information on the soils of Australia; Dr. Stanton Tuller for data on air pollution; Dr. Charles N. Forward for information on Canadian manufacturing; and Dr. W.R. Derrick Sewell for literature on British water quality. Thanks are also given to Dr. Lloyd H. Howard, Hispanic and Italian Studies, University of Victoria for translating the key of an Italian geological map; Dr. Martin Hocking, Department of Chemistry, University of Victoria for discussions on the properties of various elements and compounds; and Professor Frank Leversedge, Camosun College, Victoria for his assistance with Russian literature and for the loan of a superb atlas produced in the Soviet Union. British Columbian water quality information was also supplied by Leslie Swain and Dr. M.J.R. Clark, Ministry of Environment, Province of British Columbia. Thanks are also extended to Dr. K. Bruce MacDonald, Agriculture Canada and Dr. Thomas J. Mason, United States National Cancer Institute for computer data banks that will be of great value in the further testing of the hypotheses generated by this study. This is also true of a geochemical data bank provided by Dr. Don E. Hornbrook, Head, Resource Geochemistry Subdivision, Geological Survey of Canada. The author would also like to thank Dr. Pierre Band and John J. Spinelli of the Cancer Control Agency of British Columbia, for encouraging him to work in this area of study and for supplying British Columbian cancer data, which will be used to further explore the hypotheses suggested by this research project. Dr. S.H. Whitlow, Head, Data Systems Section, Environmental Conservation, Environment Canada has also provided information which will be of great value for this purpose; while Dr. Martha Smith, Statistics Canada gave the author several informative epidemiological articles which were of value.

Local water quality information was provided by the Director of the Greater Victoria Water District. In addition, British water quality data was made available by D.A. Woolloff, Yorkshire Water Authority; D.G. Ives, Bristol Waterworks Company; G.A. Wilford, The York Water Works; Dr. M.G. Matthews, Severn-Trent Water Authority; R.W. Brett, Portswood Sewage Treatment Works; W.O. Ord, Northumbrian Water; and F. Dawson, Newcastle and Gateshead Water Company. Water quality information was also supplied by R. Burgin, the Cambridge Water Company; K.B. Hall, the Hartlepools Water Company; F. Bell, the East Surrey Water Company; B.S. Bell, the Colne Valley Water Company; I. Burfield, the Essex Water Company; and P.A. Chave, South West Water. Sincere thanks are extended to all these individuals.

Mrs. Dorothy Grieve and Mrs. Betty Gibb, McPherson Library, University of Victoria were also of great help in tracking down obscure references, while Mrs. Sandra Smith drew my attention to certain British medical literature, with which I was unfamiliar. Similarly, the Map Library Staff at the University of British Columbia were very helpful in giving access to reference materials.

The processing of the large volumes of data involved in this study was greatly assisted by the efforts of two Geography research assistants, namely, Philip Stooke and Michael John Shasko. Philip Stooke was hired under the Federal-Provincial Summer Employment Program "Challenge 85"; while Michael Shasko received remuneration under the Work Study Program, 1985-86. Their help was of fundamental significance, as was that of Dr. Peter Keller, Department of Geography and Patrick Konkin, User Services (computers), University of Victoria, both of whom provided statistical advice and assistance and freely gave their time to help minimize my errors.

The illustrations were prepared by Mr. Ole Heggen. Mr. Ken Josephson assisted in the production of this volume. Initial drafts of the manuscripts were typed by Mrs. Jennifer Hobson Roy and Mrs. E. Lowther, while typesetting was carried out by Mrs. Diane Macdonald. I extend my thanks to all these individuals. The author would also particularly like to thank Fred Bennett, Assistant to the Dean of Research and Graduate Studies, University of Victoria, for providing computer time when required.

The work was carried out under funding supplied by University of Victoria Research Account No. 1-45725.

I should like to thank my wife, Lorelei, who by not permitting me to get away with any exceptions, forced me to think beyond the limits I had set for myself. Lorelei also assisted with proofreading, as did Susan Bannerman, who was responsible for much of the paste-up. Dr. Colin Wood, Chairman of the Department of Geography, University of Victoria, kindly reviewed the manuscript and discussed its contents with me. With all these people, I am happy to share any accolades resulting from this study. Any errors are mine and associated criticisms should be levelled at me alone.

Department of Geography   Harold D. Foster
University of Victoria   Professor
Victoria, B.C.
Canada

November 25, 1985

ABSTRACT

The group of diseases known collectively as cancer is the second leading cause of mortality in the United States. Cancer, however, does not strike at random. *The Atlas of Cancer Mortality for U.S. Counties: 1950-1969* reveals significant differences in the geographic patterns of death resulting from it. Particularly high mortality rates from cancers of the large intestine and rectum, for example, were found to occur in both males and females in the northeast and in urban centres along the Great Lakes.

Such mortality patterns appear to confirm that the causes of cancer are extremely complex. Indeed these are generally believed to be multifactorial, probably involving the interaction of a wide range of genetic, cultural, occupational and environmental variables, acting over a prolonged time period. Despite their intractability, however, these spatial distributions clearly contain many clues as to the causes of cancer and require detailed examination. A first logical step in any analysis of such mortality patterns is the search for high or marked correlations between the geographical distributions of specific cancers, to determine which cancers tend to occur together as groups, and which do not. Such similarities, or differences, in spatial patterns might be expected to indicate which cancers are likely to have a common cause, and which are not. In an attempt to identify possible spatial associations, this author analyzed data published in *Patterns in Cancer Mortality in the United States: 1950-1967*. This volume, Monograph 33 of the United States National Cancer Institute, contains age adjusted death rates per 100,000, for 65 specific or subgroups of cancers, and for malignant neoplasms as a whole. In total, data is provided on the type of cancer which caused the death of the more than 4.6 million people, during the period 1950 through 1967. This information is presented at the state scale and was derived from death certificates.

The statistical assessment of this data yielded 8,580 Pearson correlation coefficients. It is immediately obvious from these analyses that certain groups of specific cancer mortalities show marked geographical preferences, tending to occur together at high, or low, frequency levels in particular states. It is also clear that some sets of cancer are negatively correlated, mortality from one group being high only in states where that from the other is low and vice versa. A third set of relationships is also apparent, a few cancers do not correlate significantly, either positively or negatively, with any other forms, their distributions appearing to be completely spatially independent. Clearly, cancers with the same spatial distribution may possibly have a common cause. Conversely, strongly negatively correlated groups may be linked through some variable which influences both, but in contrasting directions. Finally, independent distributions suggest a unique cause or causes for the cancer types involved.

To illustrate, in white males, cancers of the floor of the mouth, tongue, the esophagus, large intestine, bladder and urinary tract organs all tend to be prevalent, or scarce, together in any particular state. In white women, breast cancer and cancer of the ovary, large intestine and rectum also peak in the same regions. In contrast, breast cancer shows a marked negative correlation with melanoma and other cancers of the skin. Where these skin cancers are common, breast cancer is rare, and vice versa. Myeloid and monocytic leukemia mortalities display very different spatial patterns, having no significant correlations either between themselves, or with other cancers. This tends to suggest that both are unique in distribution and cause.

Factor analysis was used to further examine this tendency of certain cancers to cluster. It was found in white and non-white males and females that the first three factors accounted for approximately 50 percent of the variance. This indicates that many cancers tend to have similar spatial distributions and may be linked through several common causes. This hypothesis was further supported by a factor analysis of human cancer (all four groups combined) which showed that over 60 percent of the variance in such cancer distribution could be explained by one factor alone. This demonstrates that there were many geographical similarities in the distribution patterns of United States cancer mortality in the period 1950 to 1967.

To explore this apparent clustering further, a three-dimensional diagram of total human cancer mortality in the United States was then produced. This illustrated a peak in Rhode Island and the adjacent states of Connecticut, New York, Maryland and the District of Columbia, Pennsylvania, Massachusetts and Delaware. In contrast, the lowest cancer mortality occurred in New Mexico and Idaho. Utah and Wyoming also had low mortality rates, as did Georgia, Arkansas, Alabama, Mississippi and North and South Carolina. Indeed, total cancer mortality was found to drop away to the north, west and south from the Rhode Island "peak".

In an effort to explain this unanticipated cancer mortality distribution, the author developed a computer data bank containing information on a large number of natural and man-made environmental substances, a total of 219 entries. Most of this information was derived from United States government sources, and was restricted to that collected during the period 1950-1970. Data on sunlight, precipitation, groundwater use, DDT and phosphate application, the presence or absence of dieldrin, lindane, cadmium, chromium and arsenic in surface waters, for example, was included. Information on barley, hay, potato, cotton and tobacco production was also used, as was data on a variety of mining and industrial activities.

In addition, extensive information on soil geochemistry formed part of this data base.

These data were analyzed using both Pearson correlation coefficients and stepwise multiple regressions. A large number of apparently significant links were found between the patterns of cancer mortality in the United States and various natural and man-made substances and the distribution of several industrial and agricultural activities. In summary, it was discovered that high mortality from cancer had often been associated with manufacturing and with coal mining. Very high or low concentrations of certain bulk or trace elements in the soil were also linked to elevated or depressed mortality. Of major importance are levels of calcium, magnesium, sodium, potassium, phosphorus, manganese, zinc and selenium. Elevated levels of calcium, magnesium, potassium and phosphorus, for example, were apparently associated with reduced mortality from some cancers, yet increased deaths for others. Selenium appeared to play a protective role against many specific cancers, while mercury, which probably reduces the body's ability to utilize selenium, seemed to be very detrimental. High levels of chromium were also often associated with elevated mortalities. In addition, barium, beryllium and strontium, which probably interfere with the body's capacity to utilize specific bulk and trace elements, were also associated with high mortality from many malignant neoplasms. To illustrate, cancer of many parts of the digestive tract appears to be associated with depressed levels of calcium and selenium in the soil. Mortality is especially high where sodium, potassium, manganese, beryllium and mercury concentrations are elevated. As a result, digestive cancer is particularly common in soft water areas, especially if soils are saline. This may be why states that extensively use de-icing salts contain most of the nation's highest mortality rates for cancer of the esophagus, throat, larynx, large intestine, rectum and bladder.

Since elevated levels of many bulk and trace elements are associated with high mortality from certain cancers and low death rates from others, some cancers show inverted distribution patterns. This is true of melanoma and breast cancer, and cancer of the esophagus and of the liver. Melanoma, for example, is relatively common in the south while breast cancer rates peak in the north. In contrast, unlike almost all other cancers, the leukemias do not correlate significantly with the distribution of bulk and trace elements, or with industrial pollutants, but seem to be associated with specific crops, especially hay, wheat, oats, barley and cotton. This association suggests a possible link between various leukemias and the use of agricultural chemicals, possibly herbicides.

These suggested associations between cancer mortality and natural and man-made substances were then examined on a global scale. Attention was limited to six cancers, namely those of the liver, esophagus, stomach, breast, uterine cervix, and melanoma. At least five of these, when viewed on a worldwide basis, cause very high death rates.

This global review provided considerable evidence to support the position that the spatial distributions of cancer of the esophagus and of the liver were inversely related, high mortality rates from both being rarely found in the same countries or regions. This was apparently true of South Africa, northern Japan, Nigeria, Senegal and the People's Republic of China. The only exception discovered was Zimbabwe, where both esophageal and liver cancer mortality are elevated. However, the Bantu are excessive beer drinkers and it is suggested by this author that this causes elevated potassium levels which, in themselves, may encourage mortality from cancer of the liver. Other carcinogens may also be involved.

Extensive evidence is also presented to show that esophageal and stomach cancer are very common in areas where the drinking water is calcium deficient and saline. Esophageal cancer appears associated with too much phosphorus and too little calcium and selenium, while stomach cancer is most common where potassium, sodium and barium levels are highest and selenium levels are depressed. Both of these conditions tend to occur in areas of predominantly igneous rocks. In England and Wales, for example, significantly low mortality from cancer of the stomach is found almost exclusively in counties located on, or receiving drainage from, such calcium rich rocks as the Permian Magnesium limestone, the Carboniferous limestone and the Cretaceous chalk. Significantly low levels occur on the chalk of the Yorkshire Wolds, Lincolnshire Wolds, East Anglia, the Chiltern Hills and North and South Downs. Concentrations of calcium carbonate, in water draining from such British chalk and limestone areas, commonly fall into the range of 150 to 250 ppm. In contrast, significantly high levels of male stomach cancer mortality are found in local authorities located in the Lleyn Peninsula, Snowdonia, the English Lake District, the Pennines and Tyne and Teeside. These are predominantly soft water areas, deficient in calcium but rich in potassium and associated elements, because their rivers rise in areas of shale, slate, grits, rhyolites, breccias and tuffs, all of which are Paleozoic calcium-deficient rocks. It is also demonstrated that the use of selenium as an animal food additive in Finland may have been associated with a dramatic decline in stomach cancer.

Further evidence of the association between high mortality from esoph ageal cancer and deficiencies of calcium is presented from Britanny, Normandy, Italy, Zimbabwe, Iran, Afghanistan, the Soviet Union and the

People's Republic of China. In many of these countries, mortality is particularly high where soft water is also saline. In contrast, the world's lowest age standardized mortality and incidence rates for cancer of the esophagus appear to occur in Romania, where they are 1.9 and 0.5 per year per 100,000, for males and females respectively. Romania's geology is very calcareous with chalk forming a major component of the bedrock of the Carpathian Mountains. Other calcareous rocks such as limestone and dolomite are common. Calcium rich mineral water is consumed throughout the country, which is famous for its health spas.

Evidence is also presented, by the author, to show that breast cancer mortality is associated with insufficient dietary selenium, a fat enriched diet and inadequate exposure to sunlight. This would tend to explain why crude incidence rates for breast cancer are so low in Africa, Melanesia, Micronesia and Polynesia and so elevated in North America, Northern Europe, Southern Europe, Australia and New Zealand. Breast cancer mortality is shown to be especially low in Senegal and Japan where diets are likely to be very selenium enriched.

In contrast, cancer of the uterine cervix appears to be associated with bulk and trace element deficiencies, excesses of which appear linked to breast cancer. For this reason, the spatial distributions of these two diseases appear reversed. Cancer of the uterine cervix, for example, is more common in Africa than breast cancer, while the reverse is true in North America and Europe. When mortality from these two diseases can be examined in detail, as in England and Wales, at the local authority level, this reversal is still found to hold true.

Melanoma is shown, by this analysis, to occur when iodine intake is high and diet is deficient in most other bulk and trace elements. Under these circumstances, exposure to strong sunlight appears to result in the development of melanoma. This explains why this disease is so common in coastal Queensland, where ancient soils have been enriched with iodine but leached of most other elements. It also appears to account for the spatial reversal of mortality from breast cancer and from melanoma in the United States. Breast cancer, associated with a diet containing excesses of many bulk and trace elements, is unlikely to peak in areas with a high mortality from melanoma, which is associated with deficiencies in these elements.

The global overview of cancer distribution appears to indicate that drinking water quality is a key factor in cancer mortality. This may be because the presence, or absence, of certain trace or bulk elements in potable water is a relative constant. As a consequence, individuals drinking, or cooking with, such supplies are exposed repeatedly to the same excesses or deficiencies. Such drinking water quality, in turn, reflects the geology of the drainage basins and aquifers from which it is derived, its treatment and the type of pipes carrying it to the customer. It is shown that in England and Wales, highly calcareous drinking water is associated with depressed overall cancer mortality, while saline, strontium enriched water is often found in cancer prone regions.

The author concludes with a tentative model of human cancer, suggesting that carcinogens and perhaps viruses are most damaging when trace and bulk element levels are either depressed or elevated. Indeed, it is possible that such fluctuations themselves may cause cancer directly. The part of the body in which cancer first occurs seems to reflect which of the bulk and trace elements are involved. It is also suggested that the elderly may be most prone to cancer because of the accumulation of "age elements" in their tissues, such as barium, arsenic and aluminum. In addition, they frequently suffer from shortages of vitamin D and calcium. These may be very detrimental. It is also postulated that certain cancers, such as those of the bone and testes, that have a bimodal temporal distribution, may occur in the young because of excessive exposure to strontium, which because of its chemical similarity to calcium may interfere with the normal development of bones.

In conclusion, various suggestions are made by the author for the reduction of cancer mortality. Specifically proposed is a moratorium on the use of road de-icing salts, the addition of selenium to animal feed and the revision of drinking water standards. Mercury is also apparently an even greater hazard than generally believed and requires even more rigorous control.

TABLE OF CONTENTS

LIST OF FIGURES

xiv

LIST OF TABLES

Geographic patterns of cancer are useful in developing and testing etiologic hypotheses. The rates for many cancers vary strikingly from one part of the world to another, providing critical leads to environmental and genetic determinants.

Thomas J. Mason et al., 1975

1 THE DISTRIBUTION OF CANCER IN THE UNITED STATES

INTRODUCTION

The group of diseases known collectively as cancer is the second leading cause of mortality in the United States.[1] Indeed, for some segments of the population, such as white women in their thirties, cancer is the chief cause of death. Cancer, however, does not strike at random. *The Atlas of Cancer Mortality for U.S. Counties: 1950-1969* reveals significant differences in the geographic patterns of death resulting from it.[2] High mortality rates from cancers of the large intestine and rectum, for example, were found to occur in both males and females, in the northeast and in urban centres along the Great Lakes. Males, in these regions, also suffered high death rates from cancers of the throat, esophagus, larynx and bladder. In contrast, rates for all these specific cancers were generally low in the southern and central United States. Many other cancers showed geographical clustering, including high mortality from lip, throat, esophagus, eye and bone cancers amongst females in the south and/or Appalachia.

Such mortality patterns appear to confirm that the causes of cancer are extremely complex. Indeed, these are generally believed to be multi-factorial, probably involving the interaction of a wide range of genetic, cultural, occupational and environmental variables, acting over a pro longed time period. Despite their intractability, however, such mortality patterns clearly contain many clues as to the causes of cancer. In consequence, they may be of considerable significance in the ongoing search for better methods of prevention and treatment.

CORRELATIONS BETWEEN THE DISTRIBUTIONS OF SPECIFIC CANCERS

Pearson Correlation Coefficients

A logical first step in any analysis of mortality patterns would appear to be a search for high, or marked, correlations between the geographical distributions of specific cancers,[3] that may or may not occur together as groups.

1

Such similarities, or differences, in spatial patterns might be expected to indicate which cancers are likely to have a common cause, and which are not. In an attempt to identify such possible spatial associations, this author analyzed data published in *Patterns in Cancer Mortality in the United States: 1950-1967*.[4] This volume, Monograph 33 of the United States National Cancer Institute, contains age adjusted death rates per 100,000, for 65 specific or subgroups of cancers, and for malignant neoplasms as a whole. In total, data are provided on the type of cancer which caused the death of the more than 4.6 million people, during the period 1950 through 1967. This information is presented at the state scale. It was derived from the analysis of death certificates and includes the cause of mortality identified by the International Classifications of Diseases code and the sex, race, state of residence and age at death. Members of the Armed Forces, in the United States and overseas, were also included. The monograph, therefore, contains information on the age adjusted death rate for each specific cancer, for four groups of United States citizens: white and non-white males, and white and non-white females. For the purpose of Burbank's[5] analysis, whites were taken to include persons reported as white, together with those of Mexican, Puerto Rican and Cuban descent. All other individuals were included as non-whites.

It is apparent that there was a major problem associated with the use of the non-white data in the form it was presented. This was because of the very uneven spatial distribution of this group, in the United States. For non-whites, death rates from some specific cancers were very low, in certain states. Under the circumstances, however, it was unclear whether this was because there were few non-whites living there, or because the particular cancer was rare amongst a large population of non-whites. A weighted analysis was considered and rejected, because of the difficulty in obtaining the necessary census data and the complexity this would add to the analysis. The situation, therefore, was corrected by omitting those states with a known black population of less than 100,000 in 1970, when analyzing non-white data.[6] This left 27 states for analysis of non-white mortality. With this modification, Burbank's data on the static geographic distribution of the age adjusted death rate per 100,000 individuals, by state, were initially analyzed using Pearson correlation matrices (Figures 1,1 and 2,1).

At its most basic level, this clustering approach requires a matrix of data built up of disease occurrence (or mortality) information on one axis and location on the other. As McGlashan[7] has pointed out, this taxonomic method requires that all data items within such a matrix be of comparable quality. This underlying assumption is hard to satisfy with mortality information, since its dependability varies with the number of deaths recorded

KEY TO FIGURE 1,1 AND FIGURE 2,1

TUMOR1	LIP
TUMOR2	TONGUE
TUMOR3	SALIVARY GLAND
TUMOR4	FLOOR OF THE MOUTH
TUMOR5	OTHER PARTS OF THE MOUTH AND MOUTH UNSPECIFIED
TUMOR6	ORAL MESOPHARYNX (INCLUDING TONSILS)
TUMOR7	NASOPHARYNX
TUMOR8	HYPOPHARYNX
TUMOR9	PHARYNX, UNSPECIFIED
TUMOR10	ENTIRE BUCCAL CAVITY AND PHARYNX
TUMOR11	ESOPHAGUS
TUMOR12	STOMACH
TUMOR13	SMALL INTESTINE (INCLUDING DUODENUM)
TUMOR14	LARGE INTESTINE (EXCLUDING RECTUM)
TUMOR15	RECTUM
TUMOR16	BILIARY PASSAGES AND LIVER
TUMOR17	PANCREAS
TUMOR18	PERITONEUM
TUMOR19	DIGESTIVE ORGANS, UNSPECIFIED
TUMOR20	ALL DIGESTIVE ORGANS
TUMOR21	NOSE,MIDDLE EAR, AND ASSESSORY SINUSES
TUMOR22	LARYNX
TUMOR23	BRONCHUS, TRACHEA, AND LUNG, SPECIFIED AS PRIMARY
TUMOR24	LUNG, UNSPECIFIED AS PRIMARY OR SECONDARY
TUMOR25	MEDIASTINUM
TUMOR26	ALL RESPIRATORY ORGANS
TUMOR27	BREAST
TUMOR28	UTERINE CERVIX
TUMOR29	BODY OF UTERUS
TUMOR30	UTERUS, OTHER (INCLUDING CHORIOMEPITHELIOMA)
TUMOR31	UTERUS, UNSPECIFIED
TUMOR32	OVARY, UTERINE TUBE, AND BROAD LIGAMENT
TUMOR33	FEMALE GENITAL ORGANS, OTHER AND UNSPECIFIED
TUMOR34	ALL FEMALE GENITAL ORGANS
TUMOR35	PROSTATE
TUMOR36	TESTIS
TUMOR37	MALE GENITAL ORGANS, OTHER AND UNSPECIFIED
TUMOR38	ALL MALE GENITAL ORGANS
TUMOR39	KIDNEY
TUMOR40	BLADDER AND URINARY ORGANS
TUMOR41	ALL URINARY TRACT ORGANS
TUMOR42	MELANOMA
TUMOR43	SKIN
TUMOR44	ENTIRE INTEGUMENT
TUMOR45	EYE
TUMOR46	NERVOUS SYSTEM
TUMOR47	THYROID
TUMOR48	BONE
TUMOR49	CONNECTIVE TISSUE
TUMOR50	RETICULUM CELL SARCOMA
TUMOR51	LYMPHOSARCOMA
TUMOR52	OTHER PRIMARY MALIGANT LYMPHOID NEOPLASMS
TUMOR53	HODGKIN'S DISEASE
TUMOR54	GIANT FOLLICULAR LYMPHOMA
TUMOR55	OTHER RECTICULOSES
TUMOR56	MYCOSIS FUNGOIDES
TUMOR57	MULTIPLE MYELOMA (PLASOCYTOMA)
TUMOR58	ALL LYMPHOMAS
TUMOR59	LYMPHATIC LEUKEMIA
TUMOR60	MYELOID LEUKEMIA
TUMOR61	MONOCYTIC LEUKEMIA
TUMOR62	ACUTE LEUKEMIA
TUMOR63	LEUKEMIA, OTHER AND UNSPECIFIED
TUMOR64	ALL LEUKEMIA
TUMOR65	OTHER, UNSPECIFIED SITES, AND SECONDARY NEOPLASMS
TUMOR66	ALL MALIGNANT NEOPLASMS

Figure 1.1 Cancer Mortality in the United States (1950-1967), White Males and White Females: Pearson Correlation Coefficients

OBS	_TYPE_	_NAME_	TM1M	TM2M	TM3M	TM4M	TM5M	TM6M	TM7M	TM8M	TM9M	TM11M	TM12M	TM13M	TM14M	TM15M	TM16M	TM17M	TM18M	TM19M	TM21M	TM22M	TM23M	TM24M	TM25M	TM27M	TM35M
1	MEAN		0.3766	1.1297	0.4219	0.2922	0.7432	0.3810	0.3344	0.2551	1.0860	3.3902	14.7660	0.4514	14.2552	6.4968	2.7292	9.0895	0.4500	0.4567	0.4353	2.1818	14.8583	18.0367	0.2597	0.2665	17.8402
2	STD		0.0987	0.4373	0.0802	0.1337	0.2370	0.1503	0.0797	0.1178	0.3544	1.1877	2.8426	0.0887	3.5521	2.4270	0.4048	0.7066	0.1016	0.1379	0.0728	0.6825	3.9707	5.4432	0.0654	0.0624	1.4244
3	N		48.0000	48.0000	48.0000	48.0000	48.0000	48.0000	48.0000	48.0000	48.0000	48.0000	48.0000	48.0000	48.0000	48.0000	48.0000	48.0000	48.0000	48.0000	48.0000	48.0000	48.0000	48.0000	48.0000	48.0000	48.0000
4	CORR	TM1M	1.0000	-0.3309	-0.1351	-0.1951	-0.2902	-0.1612	-0.4091	-0.2086	-0.1644	-0.3414	-0.0126	0.1973	-0.1469	-0.2095	-0.3733	-0.2502	-0.0736	-0.1321	-0.0578	-0.3351	-0.2123	-0.2606	-0.0795	-0.0886	-0.0051
5	CORR	TM2M	-0.3309	1.0000	0.3967	0.9040	0.7813	0.8994	0.4782	0.6851	0.7299	0.8858	0.2846	0.2916	0.7661	0.7153	0.3890	0.4696	0.1642	0.4400	-0.0071	0.9357	0.4020	0.6655	0.3511	0.3460	-0.0595
6	CORR	TM3M	-0.1351	0.3967	1.0000	0.2685	0.4337	0.3814	0.5627	0.1012	0.4662	0.2870	-0.2188	-0.1459	0.1746	0.0625	0.1762	0.4016	0.0964	0.1393	0.1903	0.4595	0.3681	0.3112	0.0874	-0.0074	-0.0051
7	CORR	TM4M	-0.1951	0.9040	0.2685	1.0000	0.7502	0.8544	0.3441	0.7966	0.6509	0.8284	0.3257	0.3147	0.7527	0.6868	0.2918	0.4009	0.1951	0.4423	-0.0826	0.8570	0.3571	0.5762	0.2480	0.4229	-0.0634
8	CORR	TM5M	-0.2902	0.7813	0.4337	0.7502	1.0000	0.6844	0.3970	0.5386	0.8153	0.6545	-0.0407	0.0282	0.5688	0.4703	0.0802	0.4582	0.1134	0.4852	0.0010	0.8503	0.3404	0.6236	0.1697	0.2842	-0.0564
9	CORR	TM6M	-0.1612	0.8994	0.3814	0.8544	0.6844	1.0000	0.3522	0.6904	0.6649	0.8610	0.2599	0.2599	0.8042	0.7116	0.2955	0.2892	0.0952	0.2918	-0.0104	0.8501	0.4379	0.5596	0.3114	0.2876	-0.0901
10	CORR	TM7M	-0.4091	0.4782	0.5627	0.3441	0.3970	0.3522	1.0000	0.2596	0.5168	0.3143	0.2431	-0.0939	0.0247	-0.0406	0.2824	0.4932	0.0496	0.3170	0.0376	0.5394	0.2911	0.4268	0.2081	-0.1738	-0.3618
11	CORR	TM8M	-0.2086	0.6851	0.1012	0.7966	0.5386	0.6904	0.2596	1.0000	0.5402	0.6684	0.2283	0.0831	0.5675	0.5074	0.2313	0.2493	0.1897	0.1567	0.0101	0.6176	0.2072	0.4311	0.3209	0.2816	-0.1144
12	CORR	TM9M	-0.1644	0.7299	0.4662	0.6509	0.8153	0.6649	0.5168	0.5402	1.0000	0.6198	-0.1076	0.1021	0.4343	0.3078	0.0686	0.3915	-0.0535	0.4410	0.0151	0.7943	0.2246	0.7054	0.3723	0.0610	-0.1583
13	CORR	TM11M	-0.3414	0.8858	0.2870	0.8284	0.6595	0.8610	0.3143	0.6684	0.6198	1.0000	0.5058	0.3856	0.8789	0.8477	0.3616	0.4298	0.2478	0.2894	-0.0506	0.8279	0.2082	0.5882	0.2331	0.4070	-0.0695
14	CORR	TM12M	-0.0126	0.2846	-0.2188	0.3257	-0.0407	0.2290	-0.2431	0.2283	-0.1076	0.5058	1.0000	0.6130	0.5790	0.6931	0.3358	0.1360	0.3449	0.1703	-0.0624	0.1616	-0.2165	0.0090	-0.1023	0.5673	0.3418
15	CORR	TM13M	0.1973	0.2916	-0.1459	0.3147	0.0282	0.2599	-0.0939	0.0831	0.1021	0.3856	0.6130	1.0000	0.4049	0.4049	0.2347	0.0229	0.1516	0.0202	-0.0063	0.1273	0.1197	0.0656	0.3768	0.3165
16	CORR	TM14M	-0.1469	0.7661	0.1746	0.7527	0.5688	0.8042	0.0247	0.5675	0.4343	0.8789	0.5590	0.4049	1.0000	0.9565	0.2649	0.2943	0.3002	0.2226	-0.1125	0.6985	0.1700	0.4326	0.1594	0.5262	0.2128
17	CORR	TM15M	-0.2095	0.7153	0.0625	0.6868	0.4703	0.7116	-0.0406	0.5078	0.3078	0.8477	0.6931	0.4049	0.9565	1.0000	0.2481	0.2587	0.3541	0.2280	-0.0857	0.6582	0.0713	0.4209	0.0884	0.5702	0.3109
18	CORR	TM16M	-0.3733	0.3890	0.1762	0.2918	0.0802	0.2955	0.2824	0.2313	0.0686	0.3616	0.3358	0.2347	0.2649	0.2481	1.0000	0.2715	-0.0544	-0.0285	0.0869	0.2729	0.4921	-0.1496	0.0791	0.2042	-0.1582
19	CORR	TM17M	-0.2502	0.4696	0.4016	0.4009	0.4582	0.2892	0.4932	0.2493	0.3915	0.4298	0.1360	0.0229	0.2943	0.2587	0.2715	1.0000	0.2305	0.3107	0.1398	0.5373	0.3752	0.4214	0.0868	0.1343	0.1565
20	CORR	TM18M	-0.0736	0.1642	0.0964	0.1951	0.1134	0.0952	0.0496	0.1897	-0.0535	0.2478	0.3449	0.1516	0.3002	0.3541	-0.0544	0.2305	1.0000	0.1315	-0.2574	0.1670	-0.1566	0.1879	0.0658	0.3449	0.2349
21	CORR	TM19M	-0.1321	0.4400	0.1393	0.4423	0.4852	0.2918	0.3170	0.1567	0.4410	0.2894	0.1703	0.0202	0.2226	0.2280	-0.0285	0.3107	0.1315	1.0000	0.0296	0.5355	0.0795	0.1858	0.3439	0.1840	-0.1375
22	CORR	TM21M	-0.0578	-0.0071	0.1903	-0.0826	0.0010	-0.0104	0.0376	0.0101	0.0151	-0.0506	-0.0624	-0.0063	-0.1125	-0.0857	0.0869	0.1398	-0.2574	0.0296	1.0000	0.0795	0.1535	-0.0065	0.0185	0.2012	0.1162
23	CORR	TM22M	-0.3351	0.9357	0.4595	0.8503	0.8501	0.8501	0.5394	0.6176	0.7943	0.8279	0.1616	0.1918	0.6985	0.6582	0.2729	0.5373	0.1670	0.5355	0.0795	1.0000	0.4637	0.7437	0.3503	0.2835	-0.0959
24	CORR	TM23M	-0.2123	0.4020	0.3681	0.3571	0.3404	0.4379	0.2911	0.2072	0.2246	0.2082	-0.2165	0.1273	0.1700	0.0713	0.4921	0.3752	-0.1566	0.0795	0.1535	0.4637	1.0000	-0.0201	0.1520	0.1163	-0.1873
25	CORR	TM24M	-0.2606	0.6655	0.3112	0.5762	0.6236	0.5596	0.4268	0.4311	0.7054	0.5882	0.0090	0.1197	0.4326	0.4209	-0.1496	0.4214	0.1879	0.4580	-0.0065	0.7437	-0.0201	1.0000	0.4196	0.0186	-0.0849
26	CORR	TM25M	-0.0795	0.3511	0.0874	0.2480	0.1697	0.3114	0.2081	0.3209	0.3723	0.2331	-0.1023	0.0656	0.1594	0.0884	0.0791	0.0868	0.0658	0.3439	0.0185	0.3503	0.1520	0.4196	1.0000	-0.1684	-0.0221
27	CORR	TM27M	-0.0886	0.3460	-0.0074	0.4229	0.2842	0.2876	-0.1738	0.2816	0.0610	0.4070	0.5273	0.3768	0.5262	0.5702	0.2042	0.1343	0.3449	0.1840	0.2012	0.2835	0.1163	0.0186	-0.1684	1.0000	0.4122
28	CORR	TM35M	0.1151	-0.0595	-0.0051	-0.0634	-0.0901	-0.0901	-0.3618	-0.1144	-0.1583	-0.0695	0.3418	0.3165	0.2128	0.3109	-0.1582	0.1565	0.2349	-0.1375	0.1142	-0.0959	-0.1873	-0.0849	-0.0221	0.4122	1.0000
29	CORR	TM36M	-0.0987	-0.0481	-0.0183	-0.0396	-0.0892	-0.0407	-0.0951	-0.0991	-0.2560	-0.0681	0.3079	-0.0101	0.0339	0.0225	0.0026	0.2175	1.0000	0.2305	0.3107	-0.1815	-0.1140	-0.1255	-0.0172	0.0847	0.1027
30	CORR	TM37M	0.1463	0.2041	0.5166	0.0947	0.2723	0.2881	0.0383	-0.0554	0.2499	0.1895	-0.0101	0.0389	0.2653	0.1973	-0.0879	0.0565	0.1617	0.0950	-0.1268	0.2820	0.1967	0.1852	0.0147	0.1618	0.1934
31	CORR	TM39M	-0.0174	0.4499	-0.0013	0.4554	0.1003	0.4693	-0.0617	0.1991	0.0420	0.6490	0.7547	0.5262	0.1763	0.8165	0.2648	0.2288	0.4396	-0.0796	-0.1239	0.7087	0.2005	0.5895	0.1860	0.5303	0.3438
32	CORR	TM35M	-0.3002	0.7512	0.2191	0.7057	0.4827	0.7163	0.1354	0.5106	0.3523	0.8194	0.5396	0.3400	0.8587	0.8688	0.2730	0.4011	0.3316	0.2949	-0.1362	0.5881	0.2085	0.5895	0.4003	0.5393	0.3438
33	CORR	TM39M	-0.1218	0.1266	0.5164	0.1138	0.3191	0.1036	0.5516	0.0005	0.3880	-0.1362	-0.6851	-0.4099	-0.3505	-0.4507	0.0770	0.2332	-0.0958	0.2221	0.1742	0.2406	0.4723	0.1872	0.1247	-0.3017	-0.4080
34	CORR	TM39M	0.0696	-0.1141	0.3904	-0.1622	0.2000	-0.1204	0.4256	-0.2046	0.3508	-0.3221	-0.6671	-0.3913	-0.4739	-0.6012	0.0791	0.1271	-0.3894	0.2340	0.1884	0.0767	0.3438	0.0294	0.1085	-0.4009	-0.3556
35	CORR	TM36M	-0.0611	-0.0221	0.1526	-0.0775	0.1643	0.0367	0.0686	0.1904	-0.2406	0.1094	0.0205	-0.1328	-0.1728	-0.0127	-0.0175	0.0917	-0.2795	-0.2103	-0.0262	-0.1315	0.0603	-0.0458	0.0768	-0.3611	-0.3533
36	CORR	TM37M	-0.0712	0.1095	-0.0799	0.1229	-0.0498	0.1715	-0.1472	0.2131	-0.2633	0.2131	0.3646	0.2010	0.2671	0.3112	0.3115	-0.0273	0.0942	-0.0285	-0.2533	-0.0483	0.3021	-0.2761	-0.0568	0.0768	0.0619
37	CORR	TM38M	0.0532	0.3525	0.3275	0.2770	0.4920	0.2594	0.1640	0.1440	0.5392	0.2865	0.0617	0.1273	0.2757	0.2183	-0.0527	0.2197	0.2640	0.4970	-0.0811	0.0916	0.0704	-0.5966	-0.1887	0.3176	0.1204
38	CORR	TM39M	0.1472	0.0634	-0.1404	0.2208	0.0568	0.2627	-0.3972	0.1089	-0.1916	0.1700	0.2497	0.1633	0.2901	0.3190	0.1008	-0.0284	0.4070	0.0811	0.4916	0.1496	0.0439	0.4894	0.4402	0.1579	-0.0060
39	CORR	TM39M	-0.4374	0.4200	0.2159	0.4402	0.6445	0.1303	0.0904	0.3773	0.1294	0.4195	0.1573	0.0076	0.4816	0.4814	0.2047	0.4079	0.3387	0.0862	0.0195	0.4162	0.2374	0.2996	-0.1057	0.4343	0.1221
40	CORR	TM59M	0.1079	0.1154	0.0386	0.1328	-0.1350	0.2596	0.0011	0.1499	-0.2081	0.1927	0.1955	0.0692	0.2101	0.1857	0.3237	0.0615	0.1466	-0.1287	-0.2488	0.1903	0.1902	-0.1006	-0.0138	0.5303	0.1425
41	CORR	TM51M	-0.0145	0.1716	-0.0327	0.2565	0.2905	0.0587	0.1149	0.2476	0.1349	0.2061	0.2428	0.2173	0.3667	0.4043	-0.0663	0.2634	0.3610	0.0735	-0.0166	0.7005	-0.0920	0.1782	-0.0865	0.3174	0.3411
42	CORR	TM54M	0.0310	0.3602	-0.0210	0.4224	0.3010	0.3394	-0.2295	0.3293	0.1722	0.3493	0.3521	0.6322	0.6395	0.0860	0.3148	0.0886	0.2771	-0.0135	0.3084	0.0571	0.1986	-0.1584	0.6144	0.5543
43	CORR	TM55M	0.0684	0.1611	0.1820	0.4188	0.3793	0.4015	-0.0054	0.3297	0.2830	0.3624	0.1133	0.1616	0.4027	0.4197	-0.0011	0.2303	0.1544	0.0968	0.0648	0.3570	0.1012	0.2584	0.2483	0.2132	0.1825
44	CORR	TM56M	-0.0046	0.1809	-0.0163	0.2317	0.1460	0.1613	-0.0385	0.2016	0.1620	0.3561	0.4719	0.1394	0.2692	0.2546	-0.0705	-0.0570	-0.0512	0.1399	-0.2302	0.1310	-0.1453	0.2649	0.4583
45	CORR	TM58M	-0.1472	0.4449	0.2993	0.5484	0.5125	0.4672	0.1637	0.2992	0.5946	0.4590	-0.1430	0.0818	0.2667	0.1795	0.5227	0.3896	0.2717	-0.1712	0.1089	-0.0172
46	CORR	TM59M	-0.0250	-0.2299	0.2638	-0.1290	-0.1848	0.1138	-0.2964	-0.0411	-0.4040	-0.0553	0.2025	0.1374	0.0246	0.1218	-0.0662	0.1372	0.1412	-0.0339	0.2952	0.0984	0.2675	0.1376	0.2615	-0.0501	-0.0926
47	CORR	TM50M	-0.1681	0.0370	-0.0436	-0.0057	-0.2201	-0.0771	0.0950	0.0568	0.1846	-0.1537	0.3242	0.1773	0.0344	0.1341	0.2195	0.4396	0.5484	0.1045	0.0344	0.1237	-0.0671	-0.0579	-0.1756	-0.0007	0.2510
48	CORR	TM60M	0.0321	0.0897	0.1560	0.0669	0.0985	0.1160	0.1457	0.2236	0.1229	-0.0316	0.3047	-0.0180	-0.0490	-0.1633	0.0149	0.1388	0.0642	-0.0752	0.1206	0.0983	0.2675	0.1376	0.2615	-0.0501	-0.0926
49	CORR	TM62M	-0.0846	0.2099	0.3253	0.4075	0.2413	0.3030	0.0293	0.2357	0.3306	0.3505	0.2122	0.2045	0.3574	0.3569	0.2042	0.2039	0.3955	0.1386	-0.0322	0.2547	0.2428	0.0638	-0.0497	0.2371	0.1432
50	CORR	TM65M	0.1496	-0.1169	0.2349	0.0325	-0.0211	-0.2390	0.0782	-0.3172	0.2206	-0.1931	-0.1594	-0.1840	-0.1639	-0.1843	-0.2875	0.2095	0.0586	-0.1764	0.0412	0.1491	0.5197	1.881	1.130	-0.2472	0.0997
51	CORR	TM65M	0.0038	0.4595	0.3238	0.3881	0.5479	0.4153	0.4543	0.2330	0.6901	0.2888	-0.1910	-0.0173	0.1417	0.0591	-0.2127	0.2945	-0.0283	0.4954	0.1049	0.6029	0.0903	0.5119	0.3279	-0.2013	-0.2916

OBS	_TYPE_	_NAME_	TM1F	TM2F	TM3F	TM4F	TM5F	TM6F	TM7F	TM8F	TM9F	TM11F	TM12F	TM13F	TM14F	TM15F	TM16F	TM17F	TM18F	TM19F	TM21F	TM22F	TM25F	TM26F	TM27F	TM28F
1	MEAN		0.0337	0.3181	0.2230	0.0666	0.2943	0.0888	0.1125	0.0452	0.2429	0.9271	7.7033	0.3596	15.0332	4.3966	3.4919	5.5558	0.3963	0.4123	0.2284	0.2255	2.0166	3.3599	0.0972	23.4116	8.1610
2	STD		0.0102	0.2606	0.0581	0.0344	0.1744	0.0337	0.0384	0.0292	0.0818	0.2771	1.6763	0.1001	3.0128	1.2182	0.6807	0.4011	0.0942	0.1075	0.0443	0.0685	0.5902	0.8488	0.0399	3.4962	1.6699
3	N		48.0000	48.0000	48.0000	48.0000	48.0000	48.0000	48.0000	48.0000	48.0000	48.0000	48.0000	48.0000	48.0000	48.0000	48.0000	48.0000	48.0000	48.0000	48.0000	48.0000	48.0000	48.0000	48.0000	48.0000
4	CORR	TM1F	1.0000	0.1633	0.1819	0.2390	0.6474	-0.1063	-0.0969	0.0203	0.2626	-0.0171	-0.0710	0.3756	-0.0473	0.0321	-0.2422	-0.0794	0.1507	0.1669	0.0244	0.0954	0.1713	0.2461	0.3952	-0.1392	-0.2016
5	CORR	TM2F	0.1633	1.0000	0.3533	0.9368	0.3391	0.3953	-0.0223	0.3147	0.3811	0.4419	0.1571	0.2397	0.0107	0.1669	0.0244	0.0954	0.1713	0.2461	0.3952	-0.0502
6	CORR	TM3F	0.1819	0.3533	1.0000	0.3301	0.4255	0.1117	0.0465	0.0554	0.0971	0.3497	0.1812	0.1729	0.3523	-0.2208	-0.2409	-0.0843	-0.0096	0.3000	0.0124	0.1800	0.3525	-0.1562
7	CORR	TM4F	0.2390	0.9368	0.3301	1.0000	0.3497	0.3512	0.1729	0.3523	-0.2208	-0.2409	-0.0843	-0.0096	0.3000	-0.0886	-0.0559	0.5800
8	CORR	TM5F	-0.1063	0.3953	0.4255	0.3497	1.0000	0.0111	0.2608	0.0888	0.5570	0.1640	-0.3133	-0.2481	0.3093	0.0840	-0.0401	0.3600	0.1640	0.3600	-0.1810
9	CORR	TM6F	-0.0590	0.0223	-0.2757	0.1817	0.0111	1.0000	0.1262	0.0766	0.0466	0.0640	0.0928	0.1294	0.3015	0.0770	0.3015	0.1640
10	CORR	TM7F	-0.1263	0.0053	0.3335	0.2772	0.2608	0.1262	1.0000	0.0512	0.1300	0.0890	0.1690	0.1380	0.1380	0.0880
51	CORR	TM55F	0.1820	0.0464	-0.1186	-0.0645	0.1913	0.2148	-0.0139	0.1377	0.3650	0.1899	-0.0197	-0.3518	0.1417	0.2730	-0.0537	-0.0617	0.0908	-0.3773	-0.0539	-0.0644	0.4298	-0.3551	-0.3072	0.6497	0.4298

4

Correlation matrix (male subjects):

| TM36M | TM37M | TM39M | TM40M | TM42M | TM43M | TM45M | TM46M | TM47M | TM48M | TM49M | TM50M | TM51M | TM52M | TM3M | TM54M | TM55M | TM56M | TM57M | TM59M | TM60M | TM61M | TM62M | TM63M | TM65M |

Correlation matrix (female subjects):

| TM29F | TM30F | TM31F | TM32F | TM33F | TM39F | TM40F | TM42F | TM43F | TM45F | TM46F | TM47F | TM48F | TM49F | TM50F | TM51F | TM52F | TM53F | TM54F | TM55F | TM56F | TM57F | TM59F | TM60F | TM61F | TM62F | TM63F | TM65F |

$|r| > 0.279 \qquad p < 0.05 \qquad n = 48$

Figure 2,1 Cancer Mortality in the United States (1950-1967), Non-White Males and Non-White Females: Pearson Correlation Coefficients

OBS	_TYPE_	_NAME_	TM1NWM	TM2NWM	TM3NWM	TM4NWM	TM5NWM	TM6NWM	TM7NWM	TM8NWM	TM9NWM	TM11NWM	TM12NWM	TM13NWM	TM14NWM	TM15NWM	TM16NWM	TM17NWM	TM18NWM	TM19NWM	TM21NWM	TM22NWM	TM23NWM	TM24NWM	TM25NWM	TM27NWM	TM35NWM
1	MEAN		0.1123	1.4195	0.3143	0.3677	0.7787	0.4686	0.5252	0.2716	1.2391	9.3711	24.3155	0.4071	12.3877	5.7483	3.4810	10.0475	0.3624	1.0808	0.6042	2.4830	15.5820	18.6021	0.2274	0.3373	26.9109
2	STD		0.1552	0.7424	0.1278	0.2854	0.3400	0.3827	0.4298	0.1782	0.3741	4.4226	3.4210	0.1766	3.5001	2.0514	1.4385	2.3040	0.1841	0.3971	0.2646	1.0638	6.3631	6.9338	0.1218	0.1474	5.3978
3	N		27.0000	27.0000	27.0000	27.0000	27.0000	27.0000	27.0000	27.0000	27.0000	27.0000	27.0000	27.0000	27.0000	27.0000	27.0000	27.0000	27.0000	27.0000	27.0000	27.0000	27.0000	27.0000	27.0000	27.0000	27.0000
4	CORR	TM1NWM	1.0000	-0.0216	-0.2386	0.0248	-0.3895	-0.0082	-0.0881	-0.1434	-0.1533	0.0944	0.1282	-0.2083	0.1074	-0.1298	0.2669	0.0991	-0.3661	0.1653	0.5060	-0.2952	-0.0138	0.1012	-0.5985	-0.4427	-0.5152
5	CORR	TM2NWM	-0.0216	1.0000	0.3920	0.8442	0.4959	0.7978	0.3171	0.6594	0.6368	0.8528	0.5156	0.3879	0.7978	0.7991	0.2087	0.6044	0.3358	0.1523	0.0333	0.7808	0.5084	0.7640	0.1212	0.3463	0.4032
6	CORR	TM3NWM	-0.2386	0.3920	1.0000	0.5755	0.2487	0.5136	0.3155	0.4715	0.5057	0.4439	0.1442	0.3565	0.2367	0.4242	0.0704	0.0984	0.4245	-0.0337	-0.3320	0.2674	0.1814	0.2670	0.1759	0.0229	0.3424
7	CORR	TM4NWM	0.0248	0.8442	0.5755	1.0000	0.6100	0.8328	0.4836	0.7823	0.5834	0.9406	0.6231	0.4801	0.7310	0.7982	0.3162	0.6271	0.3871	0.2743	-0.0028	0.7644	0.6043	0.7287	0.1715	0.1563	0.4206
8	CORR	TM5NWM	-0.3895	0.4959	0.2487	0.6100	1.0000	0.2594	0.5496	0.6182	0.4555	0.5159	0.2360	0.5662	0.5165	0.5739	0.1307	0.4285	0.0814	0.2671	-0.2548	0.7357	0.4667	0.4799	0.5930	0.2479	0.3842
9	CORR	TM6NWM	-0.0082	0.7978	0.5136	0.8328	0.2594	1.0000	0.1246	0.6652	0.4457	0.8811	0.6401	0.3401	0.6605	0.7758	0.1895	0.6238	0.6369	0.0712	0.1075	0.6248	0.4787	0.7358	-0.0149	0.2086	0.5714
10	CORR	TM7NWM	-0.0881	0.3171	0.3155	0.4836	0.5496	0.1246	1.0000	0.5347	0.1701	0.3187	0.2490	0.3326	0.3611	0.4431	0.5048	0.4660	-0.1352	0.1080	-0.2527	0.4085	0.4671	0.2851	0.2955	0.0391	-0.0431
11	CORR	TM8NWM	-0.1434	0.6594	0.4715	0.7823	0.6182	0.6652	0.5347	1.0000	0.4329	0.7479	0.6265	0.5662	0.6652	0.8078	0.4711	0.6364	0.3972	0.0990	0.0304	0.6124	0.5566	0.7204	0.4856	0.0975	0.3898
12	CORR	TM9NWM	-0.1533	0.6368	0.5057	0.5834	0.4555	0.4457	0.1701	0.4329	1.0000	0.4651	0.2924	0.2165	0.3126	0.3523	-0.1080	0.2106	0.2448	0.1002	-0.2541	0.5024	0.2222	0.5028	0.1052	0.2586	0.3347
13	CORR	TM11NWM	0.0944	0.8528	0.4439	0.9406	0.5159	0.8811	0.3187	0.7479	0.4651	1.0000	0.6618	0.4217	0.7777	0.8195	0.2702	0.7018	0.4209	0.2180	0.1485	0.7124	0.5201	0.8382	0.1154	0.0970	0.4795
14	CORR	TM12NWM	0.1282	0.5156	0.1442	0.6231	0.2360	0.6401	0.2490	0.6265	0.2924	0.6618	1.0000	0.1840	0.5491	0.6661	0.3173	0.5792	0.3426	0.3842	0.3303	0.5008	0.4800	0.6682	0.1440	0.0255	0.2611
15	CORR	TM13NWM	-0.2083	0.3879	0.3565	0.4801	0.5662	0.3401	0.3326	0.5662	0.2165	0.4217	0.1840	1.0000	0.5123	0.5582	0.0916	0.3432	0.2233	-0.0427	-0.3937	0.6393	0.7087	0.3146	0.2746	0.4126	0.4756
16	CORR	TM14NWM	0.1074	0.7978	0.2367	0.7310	0.5165	0.6605	0.3611	0.6652	0.3126	0.7777	0.5491	0.5123	1.0000	0.8988	0.3875	0.8057	0.0680	0.0941	0.1915	0.7590	0.6506	0.7759	0.1608	0.1018	0.3241
17	CORR	TM15NWM	-0.1298	0.7991	0.4242	0.7982	0.5739	0.7758	0.4431	0.8078	0.3523	0.8195	0.6661	0.5582	0.8988	1.0000	0.4007	0.7572	0.3224	0.1609	0.1142	0.7716	0.6207	0.8120	0.3396	0.2034	0.4468
18	CORR	TM16NWM	0.2669	0.2087	0.0704	0.3162	0.1307	0.1895	0.5048	0.4711	-0.1080	0.2702	0.3173	0.0916	0.3875	0.4007	1.0000	0.3992	0.0081	0.0943	0.4470	0.0889	0.3950	0.2295	0.1631	-0.2573	-0.3615
19	CORR	TM17NWM	0.0991	0.6044	0.0984	0.6271	0.4285	0.6238	0.4660	0.6364	0.2106	0.7018	0.5792	0.3432	0.8057	0.7572	0.3992	1.0000	0.0755	-0.1363	0.1348	0.6329	0.6261	0.7648	-0.0058	0.0446	0.3437
20	CORR	TM18NWM	-0.3661	0.3358	0.4245	0.3871	0.0814	0.6369	-0.1352	0.3972	0.2448	0.4209	0.3426	0.2233	0.0680	0.3224	0.0081	0.0755	1.0000	0.0571	0.0018	0.3071	0.2138	0.2348	0.2240	0.3146	0.5138
21	CORR	TM19NWM	0.1653	0.1523	-0.0337	0.2743	0.2671	0.0712	0.1080	0.0990	0.1002	0.2180	0.3842	-0.0427	0.0941	0.1609	0.0943	-0.1363	0.0571	1.0000	0.2580	0.1558	-0.0475	0.1370	0.2307	-0.0063	-0.1348
22	CORR	TM21NWM	0.5060	0.0333	-0.3320	-0.0028	-0.2548	0.1075	-0.2527	0.0304	-0.2541	0.1485	0.3303	-0.3937	0.1915	0.1142	0.4470	0.1348	0.0018	0.2580	1.0000	-0.1775	-0.1165	0.1819	0.0688	-0.4403	-0.3830
23	CORR	TM22NWM	-0.2952	0.7808	0.2674	0.7644	0.7357	0.6248	0.4085	0.6124	0.5024	0.7124	0.5008	0.6393	0.7590	0.7716	0.0889	0.6329	0.3071	0.1558	-0.1775	1.0000	0.7860	0.5913	0.3205	0.5367	0.6012
24	CORR	TM23NWM	-0.0138	0.5084	0.1814	0.6043	0.4667	0.4787	0.4671	0.5566	0.2222	0.5201	0.4800	0.7087	0.6506	0.6207	0.3950	0.6261	0.2138	-0.0475	-0.1165	0.7860	1.0000	0.3592	0.0975	0.3794	0.3532
25	CORR	TM24NWM	0.1012	0.7640	0.2670	0.7287	0.4799	0.7358	0.2851	0.7204	0.5028	0.8382	0.6682	0.3146	0.7759	0.8120	0.2295	0.7648	0.2348	0.1370	0.1819	0.5913	0.3592	1.0000	0.1233	0.0072	0.4563
26	CORR	TM25NWM	-0.5985	0.1212	0.1759	0.1715	0.5930	-0.0149	0.2955	0.4856	0.1052	0.1154	0.1440	0.2746	0.1608	0.3396	0.1631	-0.0058	0.2240	0.2307	0.0688	0.3205	0.0975	0.1233	1.0000	0.0809	0.2082
27	CORR	TM27NWM	-0.4427	0.3463	0.0229	0.1563	0.2479	0.2086	0.0391	0.0975	0.2586	0.0970	0.0255	0.4126	0.1018	0.2034	-0.2573	0.0446	0.3146	-0.0063	-0.4403	0.5367	0.3794	0.0072	0.0809	1.0000	0.3917
28	CORR	TM35NWM	-0.5152	0.4032	0.3424	0.4206	0.3842	0.5714	-0.0431	0.3898	0.3347	0.4795	0.2611	0.4756	0.3241	0.4468	-0.3615	0.3437	0.5138	-0.1348	-0.3830	0.6012	0.3532	0.4563	0.2082	0.3917	1.0000
29	CORR	TM36NWM	0.8306	-0.0460	-0.4165	-0.1218	-0.4629	-0.0424	-0.2462	-0.2270	-0.2146	-0.0035	0.0711	-0.4718	0.0225	-0.1765	0.3387	0.0524	-0.3083	0.0968	0.6793	-0.4158	-0.2431	0.0569	-0.5292	-0.4406	-0.6605
30	CORR	TM37NWM	-0.0062	0.0479	0.0261	0.0074	0.1086	-0.1157	-0.2406	-0.1492	0.3762	-0.0048	-0.2460	-0.0519	-0.3084	-0.3810	-0.4984	-0.3415	0.0216	-0.0587	-0.1992	-0.0349	-0.2277	-0.1447	-0.0311	0.1222	0.0485
31	CORR	TM39NWM	0.7370	0.1157	-0.2838	0.1294	0.0172	0.0202	0.2063	0.1626	-0.1600	0.2264	0.2628	0.0172	0.4477	0.2424	0.6016	0.4695	-0.3926	0.1394	0.5976	-0.0239	0.1978	0.3645	-0.2094	-0.3964	-0.4583
32	CORR	TM40NWM	0.2171	0.5413	0.2922	0.7272	0.3330	0.6678	0.3635	0.7209	0.2486	0.7569	0.7520	0.4721	0.5976	0.6565	0.4655	0.6200	0.3222	0.1916	0.1501	0.5182	0.6289	0.6788	0.0530	0.0013	0.3751
33	CORR	TM42NWM	-0.1661	0.2317	0.2745	0.2710	0.3383	0.2380	0.0141	0.4204	0.3420	0.3361	0.2543	-0.0891	0.1748	0.3352	0.2339	0.1038	0.1864	0.2266	0.2532	0.0162	-0.2610	0.5214	0.4423	-0.2801	0.1442
34	CORR	TM43NWM	-0.3541	0.1136	-0.0926	-0.0811	0.1090	0.0156	-0.4420	-0.0965	0.2263	-0.0600	-0.0564	0.1456	-0.1352	-0.0600	-0.3477	-0.3101	0.4467	0.0740	0.0185	0.2193	0.0301	-0.1666	0.2680	0.5936	0.1627
35	CORR	TM45NWM	-0.2954	-0.3839	0.3143	-0.2737	0.0185	-0.3755	-0.0666	-0.1983	0.0559	-0.4071	-0.4095	0.0756	-0.3639	-0.2796	-0.1920	-0.5105	0.0361	0.1687	-0.2971	-0.2169	-0.2281	-0.3868	0.2468	0.0028	0.0422
36	CORR	TM46NWM	0.7433	0.2170	-0.3108	0.1669	-0.1164	0.1587	0.1824	0.1270	-0.2266	0.2750	0.3094	0.0684	0.4550	0.2482	0.5546	0.5199	-0.2997	-0.0283	0.4996	0.0632	0.3730	0.3068	-0.4030	-0.2367	-0.3466
37	CORR	TM47NWM	0.7466	0.1474	0.0501	0.2881	-0.0241	0.1785	0.2700	0.3761	-0.0354	0.3244	0.3254	0.1997	0.3130	0.2359	0.5359	0.3565	-0.1395	0.0144	0.4322	-0.0351	0.3194	0.3421	-0.1655	-0.3891	-0.2865
38	CORR	TM48NWM	0.2370	0.2075	-0.0398	0.1526	0.0893	0.1040	-0.4248	0.0322	0.3635	0.1811	0.1925	0.2092	0.2086	0.1274	-0.2057	-0.1235	-0.0040	0.2618	0.2511	0.1722	0.0660	0.2050	0.0017	0.0844	0.0402
39	CORR	TM49NWM	-0.3661	0.4844	0.3517	0.5135	0.5398	0.3750	0.5580	0.4799	0.3383	0.3952	0.1608	0.6534	0.4127	0.4772	-0.0097	0.4665	0.1313	-0.1642	-0.6252	0.7166	0.6565	0.3025	0.1377	0.5844	0.5430
40	CORR	TM50NWM	0.0314	0.5650	0.2456	0.5558	0.5540	0.3263	0.7347	0.6229	0.3400	0.5183	0.3392	0.2522	0.6871	0.6417	0.4444	0.7416	-0.2337	-0.0654	-0.0237	0.4945	0.4386	0.6329	0.2056	-0.0872	0.1186
41	CORR	TM51NWM	0.0725	0.4480	0.4105	0.5789	0.3970	0.3698	0.6756	0.6058	0.2283	0.4957	0.2199	0.6100	0.5319	0.5121	0.3729	0.5737	-0.0517	-0.2724	-0.3800	0.4409	0.6312	0.4020	-0.0368	0.0600	0.1849
42	CORR	TM52NWM	-0.3845	0.3180	0.2534	0.2800	0.2854	0.4187	0.1370	0.2204	0.1466	0.3599	0.2007	0.0189	0.3281	0.4659	-0.0595	0.4429	0.1716	-0.1241	-0.1933	0.3078	0.0474	0.4557	0.0843	0.1042	0.4192
43	CORR	TM53NWM	-0.0415	0.5521	0.5279	0.5589	0.0465	0.7909	-0.0299	0.4243	0.4575	0.6147	0.4241	0.0460	0.4301	0.5341	0.0762	0.4458	0.4049	-0.0749	0.0251	0.2992	0.1421	0.6342	-0.1486	-0.0043	0.5701
44	CORR	TM54NWM	0.1855	-0.0258	-0.0615	0.1275	0.3866	-0.2527	0.6415	0.2996	0.0657	0.0311	0.0322	0.3953	0.1243	0.0256	0.2148	0.2618	-0.4386	-0.0353	-0.3623	0.1498	0.3676	0.1132	0.0502	-0.0229	-0.0663
45	CORR	TM55NWM	0.3645	0.1005	-0.0766	0.1795	-0.0189	0.2616	0.1793	0.3251	-0.2129	0.3564	0.3003	0.0606	0.3338	0.2512	0.3524	0.5815	-0.0561	-0.2664	0.1927	0.0017	0.1818	0.4980	-0.2140	-0.3423	0.1604
46	CORR	TM56NWM	-0.1964	0.3775	0.0177	0.4083	0.5666	0.2610	0.4363	0.6347	0.1768	0.3728	0.4073	0.6604	0.3785	0.5040	0.1974	0.3176	0.2857	0.3425	-0.1418	0.5544	0.4848	0.4095	0.4462	0.4067	0.2851
47	CORR	TM57NWM	0.0252	0.6494	0.3734	0.7004	0.4254	0.7282	0.4262	0.7387	0.2779	0.7921	0.5097	0.4237	0.7406	0.7825	0.3513	0.8242	0.2485	-0.0681	0.0080	0.5534	0.4669	0.8547	0.0859	0.0278	0.5458
48	CORR	TM59NWM	0.1849	0.2779	0.1173	0.1811	0.2109	0.1954	0.3154	0.1763	0.1954	0.2088	-0.0176	0.2517	0.4984	0.3465	0.0713	0.5808	-0.2896	-0.3585	-0.1465	0.2777	0.2978	0.4570	-0.2075	-0.0279	0.2007
49	CORR	TM60NWM	-0.4650	0.2781	0.4111	0.2070	0.1752	0.3323	0.0919	0.0616	0.2985	0.1818	0.0557	0.2831	0.2150	0.3052	-0.3596	0.2772	0.2413	-0.3723	-0.4929	0.4138	0.2668	0.1391	-0.0717	0.3654	0.4630
50	CORR	TM61NWM	0.2463	0.1030	-0.0809	0.0414	-0.1399	0.3130	-0.1750	0.0796	-0.1230	0.1508	0.2650	-0.1331	0.3869	0.3201	0.3094	0.4188	0.1228	-0.1089	0.5210	0.0651	0.1982	0.3227	-0.1135	-0.3118	0.0635
51	CORR	TM62NWM	0.4390	0.1538	-0.2418	0.1293	0.0172	0.0250	0.2476	0.2136	-0.1669	0.1969	0.2714	-0.0778	0.3831	0.2723	0.7103	0.3722	-0.2985	0.0656	0.5822	-0.0632	0.0938	0.2579	-0.0273	-0.4077	-0.5695
52	CORR	TM63NWM	0.5790	-0.1473	-0.3626	-0.1439	-0.1476	-0.3222	-0.0845	-0.1674	0.0386	-0.1576	0.0720	-0.2675	-0.0919	-0.2708	0.1599	-0.2071	-0.4020	0.3818	0.4234	-0.2984	-0.2431	-0.0525	-0.1234	-0.3105	-0.5898
53	CORR	TM65NWM	0.1909	0.2185	-0.0265	0.1921	0.0899	0.2054	-0.1135	0.1599	0.3892	0.2195	0.4644	-0.2925	0.1079	0.1615	0.1208	0.0912	0.1043	0.5019	0.4934	0.0231	-0.1938	0.3687	0.0841	-0.1552	-0.1426

OBS	_TYPE_	_NAME_	TM1NWF	TM2NWF	TM3NWF	TM4NWF	TM5NWF	TM6NWF	TM7NWF	TM8NWF	TM9NWF	TM11NWF	TM12NWF	TM13NWF	TM14NWF	TM15NWF	TM16NWF	TM17NWF	TM18NWF	TM19NWF	TM21NWF	TM22NWF	TM23NWF	TM24NWF	TM25NWF	TM27NWF	TM28NWF
1	MEAN		0.0363	0.3685	0.1911	0.0979	0.3569	0.1119	0.1250	0.0367	0.3290	2.1705	11.0022	0.3975	13.2617	4.6474	3.1324	6.1858	0.4110	0.9587	0.2611	0.3534	2.2000	3.9126	0.1051	22.4196	20.1227
2	STD		0.0341	0.1339	0.1085	0.0714	0.1923	0.1064	0.0865	0.0388	0.1634	0.9191	1.5030	0.2605	3.4571	1.3843	2.7803	1.2529	0.1866	0.3606	0.1270	0.2200	0.8483	1.2748	0.0840	3.4406	3.5652
3	N		27.0000	27.0000	27.0000	27.0000	27.0000	27.0000	27.0000	27.0000	27.0000	27.0000	27.0000	27.0000	27.0000	27.0000	27.0000	27.0000	27.0000	27.0000	27.0000	27.0000	27.0000	27.0000	27.0000	27.0000	27.0000
4	CORR	TM1NWF	1.0000	0.2179	0.0951	0.1098	-0.2352	-0.2002	-0.0471	0.5586	0.0447	-0.1109	0.0944	-0.1113	0.1093	0.1742	-0.2661	-0.1348	0.0719	0.1338	-0.1041	-0.0820	0.2226	-0.3387	-0.1454	0.1276	-0.1200
5	CORR	TM2NWF	0.2179	1.0000	0.1260	0.2897	0.3251	0.5507	0.3209	0.4038	-0.0330	0.7662	-0.0192	0.4397	0.7289	0.7444	-0.3640	0.4416	0.7212	-0.2858	0.0893	-0.1990	0.1522	0.1380	0.1357	0.6936	-0.5451
6	CORR	TM3NWF	0.0951	0.1260	1.0000	0.6380	-0.2067	-0.1276	-0.1728	0.1096	0.4390	0.0124	-0.1004	-0.4206	0.1813	0.4109	-0.3117	-0.0976	-0.1627	-0.1827	-0.3931	0.3840	-0.1430	-0.1618	0.7337	0.2934	-0.2965
7	CORR	TM4NWF	0.1098	0.2897	0.6380	1.0000	-0.1769	-0.0722	-0.1366	0.2606	0.4237	0.2413	-0.0401	-0.2345	0.4021	0.4815	-0.2932	0.0861	0.1363	-0.0835	-0.3555	0.5094	-0.0891	0.0419	0.3633	0.5545	-0.1965
8	CORR	TM5NWF	-0.2352	0.3251	-0.2067	-0.1769	1.0000	0.5339	0.4779	-0.1402	-0.1933	0.6984	-0.0038	0.7189	0.0032	-0.0685	-0.2607	0.0468	0.4333	-0.1660	0.1314	-0.3115	-0.2090	-0.1276	-0.0013	0.0835	-0.1024
9	CORR	TM6NWF	-0.2002	0.5507	-0.1276	-0.0722	0.5339	1.0000	0.1479	-0.0389	-0.3976	0.6189	-0.1625	0.5858	0.4835	0.5144	-0.0978	0.4680	0.6870	0.1107	0.3596	-0.0050	-0.0738	0.3247	0.1121	0.4439	-0.4049
10	CORR	TM7NWF	-0.0471	0.3209	-0.1728	-0.1366	0.4779	0.1479	1.0000	0.0684	-0.1669	0.5582	0.3179	0.6331	0.2228	0.0515	-0.0654	0.4081	0.3684	-0.1978	-0.0306	-0.3576	0.3652	-0.0675	-0.2017	0.3457	0.0475
11	CORR	TM8NWF	0.5586	0.4038	0.1096	0.2606	-0.1402	-0.0389	0.0684	1.0000	0.0115	0.1397	-0.0717	-0.0748	0.3264	0.2124	-0.2034	0.2320	0.3256	-0.0147	0.0500	0.0575	0.3072	-0.1278	-0.0631	0.3743	0.0573
12	CORR	TM9NWF	0.0447	-0.0330	0.4390	0.4237	-0.1933	-0.3976	-0.1669	0.0115	1.0000	-0.1341	0.0810	-0.5009	-0.2118	-0.0275	-0.5317	-0.5233	-0.3368	-0.2072	-0.5107	-0.1690	-0.4776	-0.3315	0.2314	-0.1194	-0.3723
13	CORR	TM11NWF	-0.1109	0.7662	0.0124	0.2413	0.6984	0.6189	0.5582	0.1397	-0.1341	1.0000	0.1057	0.6744	0.5620	0.4981	-0.2936	0.4871	0.6953	-0.2567	0.0530	-0.1173	0.1262	0.1186	0.0512	0.6376	-0.3042
14	CORR	TM12NWF	0.0944	-0.0192	-0.1004	-0.0401	-0.0038	-0.1625	0.3179	-0.0717	0.0810	0.1057	1.0000	0.0121	0.1852	0.0736	0.2445	0.2327	-0.2084	0.3550	0.2995	-0.1905	0.3335	0.2823	-0.1587	0.1108	0.0697
15	CORR	TM13NWF	-0.1113	0.4397	-0.4206	-0.2345	0.7189	0.5858	0.6331	-0.0748	-0.5009	0.6744	0.0121	1.0000	0.3718	0.1457	-0.0900	0.4182	0.7108	-0.2216	0.2041	-0.3453	0.1451	0.0890	-0.2597	0.3734	-0.0839
16	CORR	TM14NWF	0.1093	0.7289	0.1813	0.4021	0.0032	0.4835	0.2228	0.3264	-0.2118	0.5620	0.1852	0.3718	1.0000	0.8315	0.0195	0.7899	0.6087	-0.0418	0.2965	0.1336	0.4409	0.5215	0.0533	0.9043	-0.3155
17	CORR	TM15NWF	0.1742	0.7444	0.4109	0.4815	-0.0685	0.5144	0.0515	0.2124	-0.0275	0.4981	0.0736	0.1457	0.8315	1.0000	-0.2100	0.5646	0.5004	-0.0408	0.0940	0.1904	0.1983	0.3310	0.3221	0.8279	-0.5769
18	CORR	TM16NWF	-0.2661	-0.3640	-0.3117	-0.2932	-0.2607	-0.0978	-0.0654	-0.2034	-0.5317	-0.2936	0.2445	-0.0900	0.0195	-0.2100	1.0000	0.3062	-0.3103	0.4901	0.6407	0.2010	0.5481	0.6822	-0.1632	-0.1635	0.5282
19	CORR	TM17NWF	-0.1348	0.4416	-0.0976	0.0861	0.0468	0.4680	0.4081	0.2320	-0.5233	0.4871	0.2327	0.4182	0.7899	0.5646	0.3062	1.0000	0.5135	0.0259	0.4070	0.2459	0.6456	0.5806	-0.1294	0.7463	0.0252
20	CORR	TM18NWF	0.0719	0.7212	-0.1627	0.1363	0.4333	0.6870	0.3684	0.3256	-0.3368	0.6953	-0.2084	0.7108	0.6087	0.5004	-0.3103	0.5135	1.0000	-0.2178	0.1163	-0.0405	0.1080	0.0207	-0.1375	0.6760	-0.2288
21	CORR	TM19NWF	0.1338	-0.2858	-0.1827	-0.0835	-0.1660	0.1107	-0.1978	-0.0147	-0.2072	-0.2567	0.3550	-0.2216	-0.0418	-0.0408	0.4901	0.0259	-0.2178	1.0000	0.5005	0.2495	0.1453	0.3633	-0.1433	-0.1342	0.2364
22	CORR	TM21NWF	-0.1041	0.0893	-0.3931	-0.3555	0.1314	0.3596	-0.0306	0.0500	-0.5107	0.0530	0.2995	0.2041	0.2965	0.0940	0.6407	0.4070	0.1163	0.5005	1.0000	-0.1042	0.3421	0.6246	-0.1040	0.0988	0.1904
23	CORR	TM22NWF	-0.0820	-0.1990	0.3840	0.5094	-0.3115	-0.0050	-0.3576	0.0575	-0.1690	-0.1173	-0.1905	-0.3453	0.1336	0.1904	0.2010	0.2459	-0.0405	0.2495	-0.1042	1.0000	0.0757	0.2536	0.2178	0.2194	0.2714
24	CORR	TM23NWF	0.2226	0.1522	-0.1430	-0.0891	-0.2090	-0.0738	0.3652	0.3072	-0.4776	0.1262	0.3335	0.1451	0.4409	0.1983	0.5481	0.6456	0.1080	0.1453	0.3421	0.0757	1.0000	0.3576	-0.3763	0.3577	0.2683
25	CORR	TM24NWF	-0.3387	0.1380	-0.1618	0.0419	-0.1276	0.3247	-0.0675	-0.1278	-0.3315	0.1186	0.2823	0.0890	0.5215	0.3310	0.6822	0.5806	0.0207	0.3633	0.6246	0.2536	0.3576	1.0000	0.0220	0.2842	-0.0074
26	CORR	TM25NWF	-0.1454	0.1357	0.7337	0.3633	-0.0013	0.1121	-0.2017	-0.0631	0.2314	0.0512	-0.1587	-0.2597	0.0533	0.3221	-0.1632	-0.1294	-0.1375	-0.1433	-0.1040	0.2178	-0.3763	0.0220	1.0000	0.1238	-0.3533
27	CORR	TM27NWF	0.1276	0.6936	0.2934	0.5545	0.0835	0.4439	0.3457	0.3743	-0.1194	0.6376	0.1108	0.3734	0.9043	0.8279	-0.1635	0.7463	0.6760	-0.1342	0.0988	0.2194	0.3577	0.2842	0.1238	1.0000	-0.2595
28	CORR	TM28NWF	-0.1200	-0.5451	-0.2965	-0.1965	-0.1024	-0.4049	0.0475	0.0573	-0.3723	-0.3042	0.0697	-0.0839	-0.3155	-0.5769	0.5282	0.0252	-0.2288	0.2364	0.1904	0.2714	0.2683	-0.0074	-0.3533	-0.2595	1.0000
29	CORR	TM29NWF	-0.0213	0.4260	-0.1480	-0.0023	0.4921	0.2952	0.6919	0.2428	-0.2907	0.6413	0.3908	0.6990	0.4754	0.2499	-0.1105	0.5352	0.5608	-0.0704	0.1782	-0.2460	0.3876	0.0043	-0.2022	0.5132	-0.0013
30	CORR	TM30NWF	-0.1174	0.2129	-0.2186	-0.0607	0.2431	0.0734	0.4045	0.3145	-0.0771	0.2943	-0.2340	0.3375	-0.0941	-0.0910	-0.2438	0.0216	0.3669	-0.3282	-0.3006	-0.2244	-0.0132	-0.2575	-0.1250	0.0557	0.0787
31	CORR	TM31NWF	0.2791	-0.2189	0.0762	0.0614	-0.3022	-0.4003	-0.4675	0.1031	0.4421	-0.4300	-0.2926	-0.4521	-0.3398	-0.3216	-0.2644	-0.5623	-0.3209	-0.1431	-0.4178	0.0025	-0.4142	-0.3185	-0.0948	-0.3799	0.1160
32	CORR	TM32NWF	0.0045	0.5950	0.1851	0.4421	-0.0164	0.3406	0.3421	0.3276	-0.2718	0.5121	0.1429	0.3494	0.8686	0.7012	0.1535	0.8373	0.5290	-0.0841	0.2002	0.2361	0.5743	0.4836	0.0430	0.8527	-0.1364
33	CORR	TM33NWF	0.1411	-0.0148	0.0555	0.2952	-0.0013	-0.2833	0.1037	0.5392	0.1026	0.1516	-0.0020	0.0243	0.0323	-0.1735	-0.1614	0.0355	0.1891	-0.1740	-0.1441	0.1179	0.1272	-0.2933	-0.2054	0.1963	0.4966
34	CORR	TM39NWF	-0.3117	-0.0137	0.1534	0.2268	-0.2820	0.1114	-0.1029	-0.0715	-0.2703	-0.0655	0.2142	-0.1214	0.4210	0.3030	0.7293	0.4782	-0.0991	0.3666	0.5720	0.3713	0.4154	0.7986	0.3107	0.2950	0.0976
35	CORR	TM40NWF	0.3699	0.7271	0.0441	0.2684	0.0466	0.3669	0.1865	0.5689	0.0101	0.4789	0.1722	0.2467	0.7242	0.6785	-0.3975	0.5113	0.5833	-0.0415	0.0602	-0.0862	0.2148	0.0705	-0.1239	0.7049	-0.3477
36	CORR	TM42NWF	0.1271	0.3028	0.2798	0.1786	0.0289	0.4135	-0.2809	0.0082	0.0255	0.1047	-0.3399	-0.0404	0.1075	0.5134	-0.5284	-0.0155	0.3571	-0.1625	-0.1814	0.1836	-0.3528	-0.2891	0.3178	0.2534	-0.4784
37	CORR	TM43NWF	0.0498	0.3193	0.0806	-0.1985	0.5618	0.2999	0.2586	-0.0094	0.0555	0.3693	-0.1558	0.3514	-0.0814	0.1007	-0.5945	-0.1757	0.2964	-0.3582	-0.1836	-0.3015	-0.3986	-0.4453	0.2553	0.0398	-0.2771
38	CORR	TM45NWF	-0.0645	0.0355	-0.3035	-0.2407	0.5678	0.0162	0.7185	-0.0369	-0.3124	0.4321	0.2232	0.7136	0.0125	-0.2961	0.0437	0.1658	0.3162	-0.2342	0.0308	-0.3535	0.2943	-0.1959	-0.3147	0.0965	0.3454
39	CORR	TM46NWF	-0.0394	0.7500	0.2708	0.3069	0.2743	0.4855	0.2471	0.2213	0.0695	0.6178	-0.0094	0.3777	0.6534	0.7470	-0.3941	0.4533	0.6019	-0.3953	0.0575	-0.1432	0.0780	0.0916	0.3235	0.7024	-0.6175
40	CORR	TM47NWF	-0.2776	-0.2656	-0.4574	-0.3147	-0.0569	0.1375	-0.0804	-0.1735	-0.6788	-0.0978	0.0441	0.1097	0.0924	-0.1899	0.8155	0.4095	-0.0730	0.4326	0.5971	0.3585	0.4409	0.6593	-0.3679	-0.0957	0.5322
41	CORR	TM48NWF	0.4539	0.1484	0.2398	0.1294	-0.1789	-0.4238	-0.1160	0.2181	0.5097	-0.0563	0.0999	-0.1803	-0.0891	0.0404	-0.5715	-0.4240	-0.1225	-0.4018	-0.4217	-0.3907	-0.2797	-0.5025	0.1816	-0.0616	-0.3110
42	CORR	TM49NWF	0.4403	0.4052	0.1337	0.3713	-0.1454	-0.1785	0.1880	0.6967	0.0711	0.1906	-0.1367	0.0593	0.3551	0.2069	-0.3658	0.2299	0.4508	-0.3245	-0.2128	0.0590	0.2608	-0.3294	-0.0682	0.4559	-0.0109
43	CORR	TM50NWF	0.0214	0.6318	-0.0662	-0.0618	0.4768	0.7364	0.4950	0.0803	-0.4471	0.7320	0.2041	0.7067	0.6230	0.5889	-0.1312	0.6608	0.6956	-0.0179	0.2300	-0.0641	0.2731	0.2263	0.0157	0.6012	-0.3734
44	CORR	TM51NWF	-0.4664	0.1696	0.4442	0.3547	-0.1040	0.1085	0.0656	-0.3745	0.1100	0.2579	0.2796	-0.0012	0.4396	0.4977	0.2298	0.3673	-0.0212	-0.1419	0.0695	0.1754	0.1833	0.4764	0.4162	0.4057	-0.2596
45	CORR	TM52NWF	-0.0460	-0.3770	-0.1969	-0.2734	-0.4171	-0.3078	0.1239	-0.1150	-0.3070	-0.3577	0.4718	-0.1567	0.0171	-0.1625	0.8173	0.3192	-0.3610	0.3690	0.4337	0.1207	0.6403	0.5123	-0.1707	-0.0857	0.4593
46	CORR	TM53NWF	-0.2138	0.4108	-0.0376	0.1173	0.3455	0.4971	0.2985	0.1063	-0.4442	0.4736	0.0177	0.5409	0.5978	0.3129	0.2626	0.6022	0.6187	0.0047	0.4902	0.1263	0.3378	0.4127	0.0171	0.5331	0.0093
47	CORR	TM54NWF	0.4592	0.2677	0.1140	0.0774	-0.0352	-0.0469	0.0668	0.4028	-0.0263	0.1088	-0.0299	-0.0757	0.1765	0.1587	-0.1237	0.0989	-0.0291	0.1545	-0.1051	0.0529	0.2740	-0.0642	-0.0471	0.0757	-0.1929
48	CORR	TM55NWF	-0.1631	0.3519	0.2180	0.1588	0.3896	0.4385	0.1296	-0.0268	-0.0345	0.4280	0.1017	0.3048	0.3833	0.4414	-0.3170	0.3485	0.2941	-0.1781	0.0424	-0.0724	-0.0720	0.0059	0.3326	0.4547	-0.3882
49	CORR	TM56NWF	-0.2074	0.3228	-0.0799	-0.0557	0.2398	0.6960	-0.2043	-0.1408	-0.3047	0.2794	-0.2967	0.3010	0.2736	0.4015	-0.2449	0.2569	0.5002	-0.1271	0.1608	0.1343	-0.3298	0.0980	0.1016	0.2569	-0.2118
50	CORR	TM57NWF	-0.1210	0.2311	0.1647	0.1918	-0.2919	0.3465	-0.0670	0.1441	-0.4592	0.1303	0.0424	-0.0308	0.6167	0.5799	0.4918	0.7525	0.1268	0.2375	0.4236	0.5113	0.4845	0.7323	0.2433	0.5181	-0.0400
51	CORR	TM59NWF	0.5033	0.5677	0.3227	0.2553	0.1923	0.1224	0.2214	0.4701	0.2470	0.4063	0.1273	0.2423	0.4176	0.4660	-0.5524	0.1141	0.2888	-0.3930	-0.1200	-0.3814	0.0866	-0.2564	0.1827	0.4652	-0.5064
52	CORR	TM60NWF	0.0003	0.3710	-0.0936	-0.0848	0.4780	0.2875	0.6580	-0.0088	-0.1493	0.5433	0.0204	0.7113	0.2914	0.1348	-0.4094	0.3370	0.6308	-0.4552	-0.2190	-0.2482	0.0589	-0.3009	-0.1709	0.3920	-0.1390
53	CORR	TM61NWF	0.1102	0.4026	0.1222	0.1873	0.1662	0.2117	0.2083	0.3141	-0.0169	0.2280	-0.0378	0.1322	0.3398	0.2705	-0.2398	0.3664	0.3525	-0.2135	-0.0160	0.0621	0.1051	-0.0326	0.1340	0.3940	-0.1950
54	CORR	TM62NWF	-0.1604	0.3848	0.1916	0.0276	0.1937	0.3472	0.3344	0.0125	-0.1446	0.3791	-0.0143	0.3633	0.3406	0.4504	-0.3404	0.4469	0.4529	-0.4005	-0.1324	0.0773	0.0451	-0.0400	0.2610	0.3970	-0.4106
55	CORR	TM63NWF	0.1261	-0.5109	-0.1021	-0.0914	0.0395	-0.3629	-0.1299	-0.2714	0.3243	-0.2500	0.3728	-0.1854	-0.4649	-0.4356	0.1078	-0.4650	-0.5286	0.2914	0.0004	-0.1099	-0.1880	-0.0377	-0.0122	-0.4188	0.1231
56	CORR	TM65NWF	-0.2050	-0.4347	-0.2431	-0.2847	-0.2231	-0.0376	-0.3968	-0.0954	0.0236	-0.4967	-0.0213	-0.3631	-0.2935	-0.3856	0.5166	-0.2470	-0.4178	0.5619	0.4667	0.0558	-0.1677	0.4418	-0.0152	-0.4739	0.2039

TM36NWM	TM37NWM	TM39NWM	TM40NWM	TM42NWM	TM43NWM	TM45NWM	TM46NWM	TM47NWM	TM48NWM	TM49NWM	TM50NWM	TM51NWM	TM52NWM	TM53NWM	TM54NWM	TM55NWM	TM56NWM	TM57NWM	TM59NWM	TM60NWM	TM61NWM	TM62NWM	TM63NWM	TM65NWM
0.4033	0.8999	2.8686	5.0502	0.3598	0.8303	0.1048	2.4409	0.3626	1.2790	0.5396	0.7353	1.5028	0.5676	1.6426	0.0274	0.5255	0.0719	2.6297	1.9570	1.2520	0.3961	1.4986	0.7741	14.9518
0.4820	0.2963	1.2135	1.2481	0.1470	0.2138	0.0677	0.6979	0.1505	0.2267	0.1626	0.3110	0.5102	0.2718	0.4259	0.0530	0.3134	0.0558	0.8741	0.4730	0.2915	0.2626	0.4678	0.2931	2.3966
27.0000	27.0000	27.0000	27.0000	27.0000	27.0000	27.0000	27.0000	27.0000	27.0000	27.0000	27.0000	27.0000	27.0000	27.0000	27.0000	27.0000	27.0000	27.0000	27.0000	27.0000	27.0000	27.0000	27.0000	27.0000
0.8306	-0.0062	0.7370	0.2171	-0.1661	-0.3541	-0.2954	0.7433	0.7466	0.2370	-0.3661	0.0314	0.0725	-0.3845	-0.0415	0.1855	0.3645	-0.1964	0.0252	0.1849	-0.4650	0.2463	0.4390	0.5790	0.1909
-0.0460	0.0479	0.1157	0.5413	0.2317	0.1136	-0.3839	0.2170	0.1474	0.2075	0.4844	0.5650	0.4480	0.3180	0.5521	-0.0258	0.1005	0.3775	0.6494	0.2779	0.2781	0.1030	0.1538	-0.1473	0.2185
-0.4165	0.0261	-0.2838	0.2922	0.2745	-0.0926	0.3143	-0.3108	0.0501	-0.0398	0.3517	0.2456	0.4105	0.2534	0.5279	-0.0615	-0.0766	0.0177	0.3734	0.1173	0.4111	-0.0809	-0.2418	-0.3626	-0.0265
-0.1218	0.0074	0.1294	0.7272	0.2710	-0.0811	-0.2737	0.1669	0.2881	0.1526	0.5135	0.5558	0.5789	0.2800	0.5589	0.1275	0.1795	0.4083	0.7004	0.1811	0.2070	0.0414	0.1293	-0.1439	0.1921
-0.4629	0.1086	0.0172	0.3330	0.3383	0.1090	0.0185	-0.1164	-0.0241	0.0893	0.5398	0.5540	0.3970	0.2854	0.0465	0.3866	-0.0189	0.5666	0.4254	0.2109	0.1752	-0.1399	0.0172	-0.1476	0.0899
-0.0424	-0.1157	0.0202	0.6678	0.2380	0.0156	-0.3755	0.1587	0.1785	0.1040	0.3750	0.3263	0.3698	0.4187	0.7909	-0.2527	0.2616	0.2610	0.7282	0.1954	0.3323	0.3130	0.0250	-0.3222	0.2054
-0.2462	-0.2406	0.2063	0.3635	0.0141	-0.4420	-0.0666	0.1824	0.2700	-0.4248	0.5580	0.7347	0.6756	0.1370	-0.0299	0.6415	0.1793	0.4363	0.4262	0.3154	0.0919	-0.1750	0.2476	-0.0845	-0.1135
-0.2270	-0.1492	0.1626	0.7209	0.4204	-0.0965	-0.1983	0.1270	0.3761	0.0322	0.4799	0.6229	0.6058	0.2204	0.4243	0.2996	0.3251	0.6347	0.7387	0.1763	0.0616	0.0796	0.2136	-0.1674	0.1599
-0.2146	0.3762	-0.1600	0.2486	0.3420	0.2263	0.0559	-0.2266	-0.0354	0.3635	0.3383	0.3400	0.2283	0.1466	0.4575	0.0657	-0.2129	0.1768	0.2779	0.1954	0.2985	-0.1230	-0.1669	0.0386	0.3892
-0.0035	-0.0048	0.2264	0.7569	0.3361	-0.0600	-0.4071	0.2750	0.3244	0.1811	0.3952	0.5183	0.4957	0.3599	0.6147	0.0311	0.3564	0.3728	0.7921	0.2088	0.1818	0.1508	0.1969	-0.1576	0.2195
0.0711	-0.2460	0.2628	0.7520	0.2543	-0.0564	-0.4095	0.3094	0.3254	0.1925	0.1608	0.3392	0.2199	0.2007	0.4241	0.0322	0.3003	0.4073	0.5097	-0.0176	0.0557	0.2650	0.2714	0.0720	0.4644
-0.4718	-0.0519	0.0172	0.4721	-0.0891	0.1456	0.0756	0.0684	0.1997	0.2092	0.6534	0.2522	0.6100	0.0189	0.0460	0.3953	0.0606	0.6604	0.4237	0.2517	0.2831	-0.1331	-0.0778	-0.2675	-0.2925
0.0225	-0.3084	0.4477	0.5976	0.1748	-0.1352	-0.3639	0.4550	0.3130	0.2086	0.4127	0.6871	0.5319	0.3281	0.4301	0.1243	0.3338	0.3785	0.7406	0.4984	0.2150	0.3869	0.3831	-0.0919	0.1079
-0.1765	-0.3810	0.2424	0.6565	0.3352	-0.0600	-0.2796	0.2482	0.2359	0.1274	0.4772	0.6417	0.5121	0.4659	0.5341	0.0256	0.2512	0.5040	0.7825	0.3465	0.3052	0.3201	0.2723	-0.2708	0.1615
0.3387	-0.4984	0.6016	0.4655	0.2339	-0.3477	-0.1920	0.5546	0.5359	-0.2057	-0.0097	0.4444	0.3729	-0.0595	0.0762	0.2148	0.3524	0.1974	0.3513	0.0713	-0.3596	0.3094	0.7103	0.1599	0.1208
0.0524	-0.3415	0.4695	0.6200	0.1038	-0.3101	-0.5105	0.5199	0.3565	-0.1235	0.4665	0.7416	0.5737	0.4429	0.4458	0.2618	0.5815	0.3176	0.8242	0.5808	0.2772	0.4188	0.3722	-0.2071	0.0912
-0.3083	0.0216	-0.3926	0.3222	0.1864	0.4467	0.0361	-0.2997	-0.1395	-0.0040	0.1313	-0.2337	-0.0517	0.1716	0.4049	-0.4386	-0.0561	0.2857	0.2485	-0.2896	0.2413	0.1228	-0.2985	-0.4020	0.1043
0.0968	-0.0587	0.1394	0.1916	0.2266	0.0740	0.1687	-0.0283	0.0144	0.2618	-0.1642	-0.0654	-0.2724	-0.1241	-0.0749	-0.0353	-0.2664	0.3425	-0.0681	-0.3585	-0.3723	-0.1089	0.0656	0.3818	0.5019
0.6793	-0.1992	0.5976	0.1501	0.2532	0.0185	-0.2971	0.4996	0.4322	0.2511	-0.6252	-0.0237	-0.3800	-0.1933	0.0251	-0.3623	0.1927	-0.1418	0.0080	-0.1465	-0.4929	0.5210	0.5822	0.4234	0.4934
-0.4158	-0.0349	-0.0239	0.5182	0.0162	0.2193	-0.2169	0.0632	-0.0351	0.1722	0.7166	0.4945	0.4409	0.3078	0.2992	0.1498	0.0017	0.5544	0.5534	0.2777	0.4138	0.0651	-0.0632	-0.2984	0.0231
-0.2431	-0.2277	0.1978	0.6289	-0.2610	0.0301	-0.2281	0.3730	0.3194	0.0660	0.6565	0.4386	0.6312	0.0474	0.1421	0.3676	0.1818	0.4848	0.4669	0.2978	0.2668	0.1982	0.0938	-0.2431	-0.1938
0.0569	-0.1447	0.3645	0.6788	0.5214	-0.1666	-0.3868	0.3068	0.3421	0.2050	0.3025	0.6329	0.4020	0.4557	0.6342	0.1132	0.4980	0.4095	0.8547	0.4570	0.1391	0.3227	0.2579	-0.0525	0.3687
-0.5292	-0.0311	-0.2094	0.0530	0.4423	0.2680	0.2468	-0.4030	-0.1655	0.0017	0.1377	0.2056	-0.0368	0.0843	-0.1486	0.0502	-0.2140	0.4462	0.0859	-0.2075	-0.0717	-0.1135	-0.0273	-0.1234	0.0841
-0.4406	0.1222	-0.3964	0.0013	-0.2801	0.5936	0.0028	-0.2367	-0.3891	0.0844	0.5844	-0.0872	0.0600	0.1042	-0.0043	-0.0229	-0.3423	0.4067	0.0278	-0.0279	0.3654	-0.3118	-0.4077	-0.3105	-0.1552
-0.6605	0.0485	-0.4583	0.3751	0.1442	0.1627	0.0422	-0.3466	-0.2865	0.0402	0.5430	0.1186	0.1849	0.4192	0.5701	-0.0663	0.1604	0.2851	0.5458	0.2007	0.4630	0.0635	-0.5695	-0.5898	-0.1426
1.0000	-0.0284	0.7136	0.0066	0.0142	-0.2128	-0.4879	0.6975	0.5014	0.1540	-0.5596	-0.0702	-0.1791	-0.2139	-0.0535	-0.1350	0.2798	-0.2818	-0.0894	0.0487	-0.4461	0.2903	0.6731	0.5966	0.3741
-0.0284	1.0000	-0.2876	-0.1225	-0.0463	0.3767	-0.0471	-0.2115	-0.0956	0.1865	-0.0200	-0.2136	-0.1625	-0.2699	-0.1688	0.0368	-0.2345	-0.1451	-0.3062	-0.1836	-0.0202	-0.5204	-0.2905	0.1424	0.1701
0.7136	-0.2876	1.0000	0.3282	0.0875	-0.3435	-0.3364	0.8726	0.7222	0.1390	-0.2394	0.3914	0.1905	-0.1497	-0.0593	0.2999	0.5192	0.1062	0.3060	0.4089	-0.3596	0.4127	0.7801	0.5200	0.3044
0.0066	-0.1225	0.3282	1.0000	0.2457	-0.2696	-0.3159	0.4298	0.5382	0.0516	0.3779	0.4080	0.5108	0.0585	0.4461	0.3049	0.5638	0.4270	0.7145	0.1216	-0.1344	0.1388	0.2245	-0.0459	0.2076
0.0142	-0.0463	0.0875	0.2457	1.0000	-0.0379	0.0233	-0.1860	0.0628	0.1378	-0.1499	0.1821	-0.0910	0.3904	0.3931	-0.1197	0.2117	0.0576	0.3950	-0.0288	-0.2243	0.0844	0.2108	0.1087	0.4407
-0.2128	0.3767	-0.3435	-0.2696	-0.0379	1.0000	0.1165	-0.3297	-0.3385	0.4781	-0.0725	-0.4594	-0.4155	-0.1399	-0.1819	-0.4029	-0.5514	0.1543	-0.3578	-0.3623	0.1978	-0.1389	-0.2823	-0.0015	0.1127
-0.4879	-0.0471	-0.3364	-0.3159	0.0233	0.1165	1.0000	-0.5723	-0.2670	0.1013	-0.1369	-0.2218	-0.2510	-0.3001	-0.1411	0.0064	-0.4483	-0.0325	-0.3308	-0.1739	-0.0483	-0.1491	-0.4996	-0.1009	-0.0683
0.6975	-0.2115	0.8726	0.4298	-0.1860	-0.3297	-0.5723	1.0000	0.7279	-0.0005	-0.0584	0.3557	0.2931	-0.1415	-0.0038	0.2537	0.5624	0.0686	0.3117	0.3915	-0.2129	0.4034	0.6976	0.3041	0.1544
0.5014	-0.0956	0.7222	0.5382	0.0628	-0.3385	-0.2670	0.7279	1.0000	0.1498	-0.0492	0.3386	0.4197	-0.2857	0.0178	0.4337	0.5110	0.1387	0.3415	0.2706	-0.3790	0.2589	0.4709	0.3091	0.1021
0.1540	0.1865	0.1390	0.0516	0.1378	0.4781	0.1013	-0.0005	0.1498	1.0000	-0.2697	-0.1709	-0.1433	-0.2927	0.0561	-0.1586	-0.2999	0.0944	-0.1408	-0.1416	-0.0825	0.0417	0.0329	0.3957	0.2690
-0.5596	-0.0200	-0.2394	0.3779	-0.1499	-0.0725	-0.1369	-0.0584	-0.0492	-0.2697	1.0000	0.4204	0.6315	0.3343	0.1561	0.4400	0.0990	0.4792	0.4990	0.3517	0.4369	-0.2542	-0.2770	-0.4976	-0.3540
-0.0702	-0.2136	0.3914	0.4080	0.1821	-0.4594	-0.2218	0.3557	0.3386	-0.1709	0.4204	1.0000	0.6589	0.3293	0.3150	0.4799	0.3604	0.2672	0.6483	0.5912	0.1851	0.2013	0.3480	-0.1543	0.0764
-0.1791	-0.1625	0.1905	0.5108	-0.0910	-0.4155	-0.2510	0.2931	0.4197	-0.1433	0.6315	0.6589	1.0000	0.1885	0.2312	0.6222	0.4017	0.3148	0.6033	0.4180	0.2283	-0.0727	0.1816	-0.2060	-0.4436
-0.2139	-0.2699	-0.1497	0.0585	0.3904	-0.1399	-0.3001	-0.1415	-0.2857	-0.2927	0.3343	0.3293	0.1885	1.0000	0.4982	-0.2050	0.2179	-0.0518	0.5129	0.3523	0.5490	0.2532	-0.0326	-0.5257	-0.0428
-0.0535	-0.1688	-0.0593	0.4461	0.3931	-0.1819	-0.1411	-0.0038	0.0178	0.0561	0.1561	0.3150	0.2312	0.4982	1.0000	-0.2980	0.3179	-0.0974	0.6714	0.3079	0.3185	0.3895	-0.1065	-0.2865	0.2124
-0.1350	0.0368	0.2999	0.3049	-0.1197	-0.4029	0.0064	0.2537	0.4337	-0.1586	0.4400	0.4799	0.6222	-0.2050	-0.2980	1.0000	0.3583	0.3888	0.2517	0.3312	-0.2110	-0.3358	0.0941	0.1867	-0.2721
0.2798	-0.2345	0.5192	0.5638	0.2117	-0.5514	-0.4483	0.5624	0.5110	-0.2999	0.0990	0.3604	0.4017	0.2179	0.3179	0.3583	1.0000	0.0438	0.6873	0.4270	-0.1879	0.3455	0.3066	0.0166	-0.0880
-0.2818	-0.1451	0.1062	0.4270	0.0576	0.1543	-0.0325	0.0686	0.1387	0.0944	0.4792	0.2672	0.3148	-0.0518	-0.0974	0.3888	0.0438	1.0000	0.3548	0.0235	-0.0022	-0.1742	0.0762	-0.0426	0.0978
-0.0894	-0.3062	0.3060	0.7145	0.3950	-0.3578	-0.3308	0.3117	0.3415	-0.1408	0.4990	0.6483	0.6033	0.5129	0.6714	0.2517	0.6873	0.3548	1.0000	0.5494	0.1645	0.2911	0.1683	-0.2499	0.0109
0.0487	-0.1836	0.4089	0.1216	-0.0288	-0.3623	-0.1739	0.3915	0.2706	-0.1416	0.3517	0.5912	0.4180	0.3523	0.3079	0.3312	0.4270	0.0235	0.5494	1.0000	0.3525	0.4024	0.1082	-0.0846	-0.0752
-0.4461	-0.0202	-0.3596	-0.1344	-0.2243	0.1978	-0.0483	-0.2129	-0.3790	-0.0825	0.4369	0.1851	0.2283	0.5490	0.3185	-0.2110	-0.1879	-0.0022	0.1645	0.3525	1.0000	0.0894	-0.2754	-0.5960	-0.1684
0.2903	-0.5204	0.4127	0.1388	0.0844	-0.1389	-0.1491	0.4034	0.2589	0.0417	-0.2542	0.2013	-0.0727	0.2532	0.3895	-0.3358	0.3455	-0.1742	0.2911	0.4024	0.0894	1.0000	0.2069	-0.0987	0.1654
0.6731	-0.2905	0.7801	0.2245	0.2108	-0.2823	-0.4996	0.6976	0.4709	0.0329	-0.2770	0.3480	0.1816	-0.0326	-0.1065	0.0941	0.3066	0.0762	0.1683	0.1082	-0.2754	0.2069	1.0000	0.4405	0.3083
0.5966	0.1424	0.5200	-0.0459	0.1087	-0.0015	-0.1009	0.3041	0.3091	0.3957	-0.4976	-0.1543	-0.2060	-0.5257	-0.2865	0.1867	0.0166	-0.0426	-0.2499	-0.0846	-0.5960	-0.0987	0.4405	1.0000	0.3710
0.3741	0.1701	0.3044	0.2076	0.4407	0.1127	-0.0683	0.1544	0.1021	0.2690	-0.3540	0.0764	-0.4436	-0.0428	0.2124	-0.2721	-0.0880	0.0978	0.0109	-0.0752	-0.1684	0.1654	0.3083	0.3710	1.0000

TM29NWF	TM30NWF	TM31NWF	TM32NWF	TM33NWF	TM39NWF	TM40NWF	TM42NWF	TM43NWF	TM45NWF	TM46NWF	TM47NWF	TM48NWF	TM49NWF	TM50NWF	TM51NWF	TM52NWF	TM53NWF	TM54NWF	TM55NWF	TM56NWF	TM57NWF	TM59NWF	TM60NWF	TM61NWF	TM62NWF	TM63NWF	TM65NWF
1.8255	0.1849	10.1305	6.5546	0.9844	1.5272	3.0711	0.2719	0.6122	0.1067	1.4666	0.8056	0.8453	0.4515	0.3500	0.8839	0.3362	0.8551	0.0140	0.2872	0.0472	1.8024	0.9572	0.9200	0.2867	1.0214	0.5578	13.5114
0.9896	0.1288	2.5897	1.2849	0.2178	0.4716	0.8613	0.1142	0.2006	0.1522	0.4634	0.4263	0.3140	0.2220	0.1956	0.3397	0.1757	0.2809	0.0190	0.1110	0.0459	0.5474	0.2693	0.3153	0.1568	0.2679	0.1891	3.0980
27.0000	27.0000	27.0000	27.0000	27.0000	27.0000	27.0000	27.0000	27.0000	27.0000	27.0000	27.0000	27.0000	27.0000	27.0000	27.0000	27.0000	27.0000	27.0000	27.0000	27.0000	27.0000	27.0000	27.0000	27.0000	27.0000	27.0000	27.0000
-0.0213	-0.1174	0.2791	0.0045	0.1411	-0.3117	0.3699	0.1271	0.0498	-0.0645	-0.0394	-0.2776	0.4539	0.4403	0.0214	-0.4664	-0.0460	-0.2138	0.4592	-0.1631	-0.2074	-0.1210	0.5033	0.0003	0.1102	-0.1604	0.1261	-0.2050
0.4260	0.2129	-0.2189	0.5950	-0.0148	-0.0137	0.7271	0.3028	0.3193	0.0355	0.7500	-0.2656	0.1484	0.4052	0.6318	0.1696	-0.3770	0.4108	0.2677	0.3519	0.3228	0.2311	0.5677	0.3710	0.4026	0.3848	-0.5109	-0.4347
-0.1480	-0.2186	0.0762	0.1851	0.0555	0.1534	0.0441	0.2798	0.0806	-0.3035	0.2708	-0.4574	0.2398	0.1337	-0.0662	0.4442	-0.1969	-0.0376	0.1140	0.2180	-0.0799	0.1647	0.3227	-0.0936	0.1222	0.1916	-0.1021	-0.2431
-0.0023	-0.0607	0.0614	0.4421	0.2952	0.2268	0.2684	0.1786	-0.1985	-0.2407	0.3069	-0.3147	0.1294	0.3713	-0.0618	0.3547	-0.2734	0.1173	0.0774	0.1588	-0.0557	0.1918	0.2553	-0.0848	0.1873	0.0276	-0.0914	-0.2847
0.4921	0.2431	-0.3022	-0.0164	-0.0013	-0.2820	0.0466	0.0289	0.5618	0.5678	0.2743	-0.0569	-0.1789	-0.1454	0.4768	-0.1040	-0.4171	0.3455	-0.0352	0.3896	0.2398	-0.2919	0.1923	0.4780	0.1662	0.1937	0.0395	-0.2231
0.2952	0.0734	-0.4003	0.3406	-0.2833	0.1114	0.3669	0.4135	0.2999	0.0162	0.4855	0.1375	-0.4238	-0.1785	0.7364	0.1085	-0.3078	0.4971	-0.0469	0.4385	0.6960	0.3465	0.1224	0.2875	0.2117	0.3472	-0.3629	-0.0376
0.6919	0.4045	-0.4675	0.3421	0.1037	-0.1029	0.1865	-0.2809	0.2586	0.7185	0.2471	-0.0804	-0.1160	0.1880	0.4950	0.0656	0.1239	0.2985	0.0668	0.1296	-0.2043	-0.0670	0.2214	0.6580	0.2083	0.3344	-0.1299	-0.3968
0.2428	0.3145	0.1031	0.3276	0.5392	-0.0715	0.5689	0.0082	-0.0094	-0.0369	0.2213	-0.1735	0.2181	0.6967	0.0803	-0.3745	-0.1150	0.1063	0.4028	-0.0268	-0.1408	0.1441	0.4701	-0.0088	0.3141	0.0125	-0.2714	-0.0954
-0.2907	-0.0771	0.4421	-0.2718	0.1026	-0.2703	0.0101	0.0255	0.0555	-0.3124	0.0695	-0.6788	0.5097	0.0711	-0.4471	0.1100	-0.3070	-0.4442	-0.0263	-0.0345	-0.3047	-0.4592	0.2470	-0.1493	-0.0169	-0.1446	0.3243	0.0236
0.6413	0.2943	-0.4300	0.5121	0.1516	-0.0655	0.4789	0.1047	0.3693	0.4321	0.6178	-0.0978	-0.0563	0.1906	0.7320	0.2579	-0.3577	0.4736	0.1088	0.4280	0.2794	0.1303	0.4063	0.5433	0.2280	0.3791	-0.2500	-0.4967
0.3908	-0.2340	-0.2926	0.1429	-0.0020	0.2142	0.1722	-0.3399	-0.1558	0.2232	-0.0094	0.0441	0.0999	-0.1367	0.2041	0.2796	0.4718	0.0177	-0.0299	0.1017	-0.2967	0.0424	0.1273	0.0204	-0.0378	-0.0143	0.3728	-0.0213
0.6990	0.3375	-0.4521	0.3494	0.0243	-0.1214	0.2467	-0.0404	0.3514	0.7136	0.3777	0.1097	-0.1803	0.0593	0.7067	-0.0012	-0.1567	0.5409	-0.0757	0.3048	0.3010	-0.0308	0.2423	0.7113	0.1322	0.3633	-0.1854	-0.3631
0.4754	-0.0941	-0.3398	0.8686	0.0323	0.4210	0.7242	0.1075	-0.0814	0.0125	0.6534	0.0924	-0.0891	0.3551	0.6230	0.4396	0.0171	0.5978	0.1765	0.3833	0.2736	0.6167	0.4176	0.2914	0.3398	0.3406	-0.4649	-0.2935
0.2499	-0.0910	-0.3216	0.7012	-0.1735	0.3030	0.6785	0.5134	0.1007	-0.2961	0.7470	-0.1899	0.0404	0.2069	0.5889	0.4977	-0.1625	0.3129	0.1587	0.4414	0.4015	0.5799	0.4660	0.1348	0.2705	0.4504	-0.4356	-0.3856
-0.1105	-0.2438	-0.2644	0.1535	-0.1614	0.7293	-0.3975	-0.5284	-0.5945	0.0437	-0.3941	0.8155	-0.5715	-0.3658	-0.1312	0.2298	0.8173	0.2626	-0.1237	-0.3170	-0.2449	0.4918	-0.5524	-0.4094	-0.2398	-0.3404	0.1078	0.5166
0.5352	0.0216	-0.5623	0.8373	0.0355	0.4782	0.5113	-0.0155	-0.1757	0.1658	0.4533	0.4095	-0.4240	0.2299	0.6608	0.3673	0.3192	0.6022	0.0989	0.3485	0.2569	0.7525	0.1141	0.3370	0.3664	0.4469	-0.4650	-0.2470
0.5608	0.3669	-0.3209	0.5290	0.1891	-0.0991	0.5833	0.3571	0.2964	0.3162	0.6019	-0.0730	-0.1225	0.4508	0.6956	-0.0212	-0.3610	0.6187	-0.0291	0.2941	0.5002	0.1268	0.2888	0.6308	0.3525	0.4529	-0.5286	-0.4178
-0.0704	-0.3282	-0.1431	-0.0841	-0.1740	0.3666	-0.0415	-0.1625	-0.3582	-0.2342	-0.3953	0.4326	-0.4018	-0.3245	-0.0179	-0.1419	0.3690	0.0047	0.1545	-0.1781	-0.1271	0.2375	-0.3930	-0.4552	-0.2135	-0.4005	0.2914	0.5619
0.1782	-0.3006	-0.4178	0.2002	-0.1441	0.5720	0.0602	-0.1814	-0.1836	0.0308	0.0575	0.5971	-0.4217	-0.2128	0.2300	0.0695	0.4337	0.4902	-0.1051	0.0424	0.1608	0.4236	-0.1200	-0.2190	-0.0160	-0.1324	0.0004	0.4667
-0.2460	-0.2244	0.0025	0.2361	0.1179	0.3713	-0.0862	0.1836	-0.3015	-0.3535	-0.1432	0.3585	-0.3907	0.0590	-0.0641	0.1754	0.1207	0.1263	0.0529	-0.0724	0.1343	0.5113	-0.3814	-0.2482	0.0621	0.0773	-0.1099	0.0558
0.3876	-0.0132	-0.4142	0.5743	0.1272	0.4154	0.2148	-0.3528	-0.3986	0.2943	0.0780	0.4409	-0.2797	0.2608	0.2731	0.1833	0.6403	0.3378	0.2740	-0.0720	-0.3298	0.4845	0.0866	0.0589	0.1051	0.0451	-0.1880	-0.1677
0.0043	-0.2575	-0.3185	0.4836	-0.2933	0.7986	0.0705	-0.2891	-0.4453	-0.1959	0.0916	0.6593	-0.5025	-0.3294	0.2263	0.4764	0.5123	0.4127	-0.0642	0.0059	0.0980	0.7323	-0.2564	-0.3009	-0.0326	-0.0400	-0.0377	0.4418
-0.2022	-0.1250	-0.0948	0.0430	-0.2054	0.3107	-0.1239	0.3178	0.2553	-0.3147	0.3235	-0.3679	0.1816	-0.0682	0.0157	0.4162	-0.1707	0.0171	-0.0471	0.3326	0.1016	0.2433	0.1827	-0.1709	0.1340	0.2610	-0.0122	-0.0152
0.5132	0.0557	-0.3799	0.8527	0.1963	0.2950	0.7049	0.2534	0.0398	0.0965	0.7024	-0.0957	-0.0616	0.4559	0.6012	0.4057	-0.0857	0.5331	0.0757	0.4547	0.2569	0.5181	0.4652	0.3920	0.3940	0.3970	-0.4188	-0.4739
-0.0013	0.0787	0.1160	-0.1364	0.4966	0.0976	-0.3477	-0.4784	-0.2771	0.3454	-0.6175	0.5322	-0.3110	-0.0109	-0.3734	-0.2596	0.4593	0.0093	-0.1929	-0.3882	-0.2118	-0.0400	-0.5064	-0.1390	-0.1950	-0.4106	0.1231	0.2039
1.0000	0.3616	-0.6115	0.5350	0.2889	-0.0001	0.4692	-0.1191	0.2034	0.6875	0.4955	-0.0819	-0.0110	0.3524	0.7041	0.1659	-0.0470	0.5339	0.1342	0.4323	-0.0282	0.0355	0.3960	0.6641	0.2169	0.4926	-0.2222	-0.5172
0.3616	1.0000	-0.0805	0.0871	0.3501	-0.2974	0.1610	-0.0326	0.1557	0.3773	0.1406	-0.2507	0.0317	0.2241	0.1586	-0.1693	-0.2138	0.0457	-0.0914	0.0078	-0.0739	-0.2419	0.0686	0.2821	0.0756	0.2301	-0.2300	-0.2572
-0.6115	-0.0805	1.0000	-0.4409	0.0965	-0.4431	-0.0773	-0.0875	-0.0052	-0.3184	-0.4192	-0.2043	0.3271	-0.0024	-0.6375	-0.4212	-0.2714	-0.4998	0.1180	-0.3849	-0.0891	-0.4397	-0.0437	-0.2493	-0.0775	-0.5210	0.1882	0.2146
0.5350	0.0871	-0.4409	1.0000	0.0833	0.5096	0.5534	0.0028	-0.2404	0.1213	0.6082	0.1081	-0.2320	0.3631	0.5712	0.5112	0.1658	0.6233	0.1983	0.3692	0.0736	0.6581	0.3302	0.3251	0.4077	0.4130	-0.4657	-0.4115
0.2889	0.3501	0.0965	0.0833	1.0000	-0.2192	0.1779	-0.2323	-0.1028	0.3898	-0.1029	-0.0639	0.2451	0.5141	-0.1212	-0.1807	-0.0387	0.0478	-0.1459	-0.1221	-0.1383	-0.1886	0.1713	0.1414	-0.0684	-0.1361	0.0377	-0.2137
-0.0001	-0.2974	-0.4431	0.5096	-0.2192	1.0000	-0.1141	-0.2131	-0.5046	-0.1840	0.1458	0.4777	-0.4923	-0.1541	0.0419	0.5999	0.5894	0.4775	-0.1113	0.0513	-0.1025	0.7262	-0.2257	-0.3808	0.0371	-0.0057	-0.0675	0.3531
0.4692	0.1610	-0.0773	0.5534	0.1779	-0.1141	1.0000	0.2763	0.1423	-0.0827	0.5691	-0.2565	0.2036	0.5231	0.5146	-0.0556	-0.2626	0.1949	0.3451	0.4907	0.2785	0.2284	0.5382	0.2989	0.5146	0.2992	-0.4030	-0.3936
-0.1191	-0.0326	-0.0875	0.0028	-0.2323	-0.2131	0.2763	1.0000	0.4820	-0.4493	0.4770	-0.4115	0.1107	0.0735	0.2665	-0.0020	-0.5150	-0.0890	-0.1463	0.3972	0.6684	0.0897	0.2187	0.0618	0.2084	0.4328	-0.3828	-0.3443
0.2034	0.1557	-0.0052	-0.2404	-0.1028	-0.5046	0.1423	0.4820	1.0000	0.1551	0.4032	-0.4542	0.3057	0.0180	0.2990	-0.2069	-0.5513	-0.1501	-0.0068	0.3127	0.3714	-0.3068	0.3567	0.3576	0.0692	0.3259	-0.1095	-0.3057
0.6875	0.3773	-0.3184	0.1213	0.3898	-0.1840	-0.0827	-0.4493	0.1551	1.0000	0.0075	0.0604	-0.0416	0.1532	0.3272	-0.0190	0.1066	0.3902	-0.1224	0.0343	-0.2331	-0.3338	0.1465	0.6528	-0.0295	0.1195	0.1239	-0.3665
0.4955	0.1406	-0.4192	0.6082	-0.1029	0.1458	0.5691	0.4770	0.4032	0.0075	1.0000	-0.4309	0.1498	0.3282	0.5763	0.4471	-0.3430	0.3953	0.0895	0.6078	0.3221	0.2657	0.6420	0.3771	0.3874	0.6526	-0.4027	-0.5134
-0.0819	-0.2507	-0.2043	0.1081	-0.0639	0.4777	-0.2565	-0.4115	-0.4542	0.0604	-0.4309	1.0000	-0.6703	-0.3084	0.0324	0.0014	0.5486	0.3162	-0.0456	-0.3216	0.0795	0.4966	-0.6079	-0.2478	-0.2259	-0.2613	-0.0288	0.4751
-0.0110	0.0317	0.3271	-0.2320	0.2451	-0.4923	0.2036	0.1107	0.3057	-0.0416	0.1498	-0.6703	1.0000	0.3568	-0.1413	-0.0969	-0.3208	-0.4889	0.1424	0.0190	-0.1621	-0.3904	0.5503	0.1037	-0.1453	0.0356	0.2008	-0.3517
0.3524	0.2241	-0.0024	0.3631	0.5141	-0.1541	0.5231	0.0735	0.0180	0.1532	0.3282	-0.3084	0.3568	1.0000	0.1038	-0.2203	-0.1889	0.2358	0.3274	0.1099	-0.1499	-0.0194	0.3786	0.3809	0.4878	0.2661	-0.3639	-0.4577
0.7041	0.1586	-0.6375	0.5712	-0.1212	0.0419	0.5146	0.2665	0.2990	0.3272	0.5763	0.0324	-0.1413	0.1038	1.0000	0.2449	-0.1080	0.5386	0.1277	0.4976	0.3914	0.3696	0.3369	0.6264	0.2550	0.6514	-0.3486	-0.4441
0.1659	-0.1693	-0.4212	0.5112	-0.1807	0.5999	-0.0556	-0.0020	-0.2069	-0.0190	0.4471	0.0014	-0.0969	-0.2203	0.2449	1.0000	0.2424	0.3357	-0.2449	0.2410	0.0021	0.4348	0.0601	0.0431	-0.1061	0.3479	-0.0702	-0.1956
-0.0470	-0.2138	-0.2714	0.1658	-0.0387	0.5894	-0.2626	-0.5150	-0.5513	0.1066	-0.3430	0.5486	-0.3208	-0.1889	-0.1080	0.2424	1.0000	0.0837	-0.1518	-0.2753	-0.3950	0.3990	-0.3520	-0.2546	-0.0976	-0.1588	0.2686	0.3223
0.5339	0.0457	-0.4998	0.6233	0.0478	0.4775	0.1949	-0.0890	-0.1501	0.3902	0.3953	0.3162	-0.4889	0.2358	0.5386	0.3357	0.0837	1.0000	-0.0897	0.2280	0.1394	0.3223	0.0173	0.4297	0.3519	0.3459	-0.3776	-0.0796
0.1342	-0.0914	0.1180	0.1983	-0.1459	-0.1113	0.3451	-0.1463	-0.0068	-0.1224	0.0895	-0.0456	0.1424	0.3274	0.1277	-0.2449	-0.1518	-0.0897	1.0000	0.0192	-0.2959	0.1433	0.2872	0.0271	0.2165	0.0539	-0.0834	-0.1569
0.4323	0.0078	-0.3849	0.3692	-0.1221	0.0513	0.4907	0.3972	0.3127	0.0343	0.6078	-0.3216	0.0190	0.1099	0.4976	0.2410	-0.2753	0.2280	0.0192	1.0000	0.3211	0.1842	0.4017	0.3167	0.5984	0.4592	-0.1794	-0.4442
-0.0282	-0.0739	-0.0891	0.0736	-0.1383	-0.1025	0.2785	0.6684	0.3714	-0.2331	0.3221	0.0795	-0.1621	-0.1499	0.3914	0.0021	-0.3950	0.1394	-0.2959	0.3211	1.0000	0.2388	0.0237	0.1433	0.0982	0.3274	-0.4586	-0.1329
0.0355	-0.2419	-0.4397	0.6581	-0.1886	0.7262	0.2284	0.0897	-0.3068	-0.3338	0.2657	0.4966	-0.3904	-0.0194	0.3696	0.4348	0.3990	0.3223	0.1433	0.1842	0.2388	1.0000	-0.0607	-0.2036	0.1193	0.2351	-0.3603	0.0829
0.3960	0.0686	-0.0437	0.3302	0.1713	-0.2257	0.5382	0.2187	0.3567	0.1465	0.6420	-0.6079	0.5503	0.3786	0.3369	0.0601	-0.3520	0.0173	0.2872	0.4017	0.0237	-0.0607	1.0000	0.2960	0.2307	0.2901	-0.0396	-0.5348
0.6641	0.2821	-0.2493	0.3251	0.1414	-0.3808	0.2989	0.0618	0.3576	0.6528	0.3771	-0.2478	0.1037	0.3809	0.6264	0.0431	-0.2546	0.4297	0.0271	0.3167	0.1433	-0.2036	0.2960	1.0000	0.3289	0.5916	-0.2632	-0.6484
0.2169	0.0756	-0.0775	0.4077	-0.0684	0.0371	0.5146	0.2084	0.0692	-0.0295	0.3874	-0.2259	-0.1453	0.4878	0.2550	-0.1061	-0.0976	0.3519	0.2165	0.5984	0.0982	0.1193	0.2307	0.3289	1.0000	0.3804	-0.3380	-0.3028
0.4926	0.2301	-0.5210	0.4130	-0.1361	-0.0057	0.2992	0.4328	0.3259	0.1195	0.6526	-0.2613	0.0356	0.2661	0.6514	0.3479	-0.1588	0.3459	0.0539	0.4592	0.3274	0.2351	0.2901	0.5916	0.3804	1.0000	-0.4152	-0.5567
-0.2222	-0.2300	0.1882	-0.4657	0.0377	-0.0675	-0.4030	-0.3828	-0.1095	0.1239	-0.4027	-0.0288	0.2008	-0.3639	-0.3486	-0.0702	0.2686	-0.3776	-0.0834	-0.1794	-0.4586	-0.3603	-0.0396	-0.2632	-0.3380	-0.4152	1.0000	0.3049
-0.5172	-0.2572	0.2146	-0.4115	-0.2137	0.3531	-0.3936	-0.3443	-0.3057	-0.3665	-0.5134	0.4751	-0.3517	-0.4577	-0.4441	-0.1956	0.3223	-0.0796	-0.1569	-0.4442	-0.1329	0.0829	-0.5348	-0.6484	-0.3028	-0.5567	0.3049	1.0000

$|r| > 0.369 \quad p < 0.05 \quad n = 27$

and the population size involved, as well as with the quality of diagnosis. Random fluctuations probably reduce confidence when small numbers are involved. Since this particular analysis involves what is almost certainly one of the largest samples ever analyzed in this manner (4.6 million mortalities), the impact of this problem is minimized.

It has also been suggested that data used to derive such Pearson correlation matrices be subjected to stochastic tests to ascertain which localities deviate, at selected significant levels in either tail of the distribution, that is in a high (above normal) or low (below normal) manner from national or regional norms.[8] Fortunately, such an analysis had already been carried out on a very similar data set by Mason et al.[9] who used such United States mortality information to produce the *Atlas of Mortality for U.S. Counties: 1950-1969*. Maps are available, therefore, for the 48 contiguous states, which show the spatial variations of mortality, on a county, or state economic area basis. These illustrations indicate whether a particular region has a significantly high (in the highest decile), or significantly low, age adjusted death rate from different specific cancers. Burbank[10] has also produced similar maps, at the state scale, for all the data sets used by the present author. It was possible, therefore, to visually check variations of specific cancers, or groups of cancers, from the national or regional norms using these atlases of mortality. Since such significance testing has already been conducted twice this step was omitted here.[11]

With these limitations in mind, the Pearson correlation matrices were examined to see which specific cancers, or groups of cancers, exhibited locational similarities or dissimilarities, when viewed over the contiguous United States (Figures 1,1 and 2,1). It should be stressed, however, that because of the uneven distribution of the non-whites in the United States, related correlations are less valid than for whites. Figures 1,1 and 2,1 show each correlation twice, since, for example, the relationship between cancer of the tongue and the esophagus is the same as that between the esophagus and the tongue. Normally, therefore, such Pearson correlation matrices are truncated and only one-half is presented.[12] However, those generated by this study are so large that this technique makes them very difficult to read. For this reason they are presented complete. The author is fully aware that, at their reduced scale, they are still very hard on the eye. However, financial constraints left two options, to publish them at this scale, or not to provide them at all. Since the reduction of the death rate is a unifying goal for workers in this area, the author would be happy to supply enlarged copies, or the information on computer tape, to anyone wishing to further explore these relationships.

It is immediately obvious from these figures that certain groups of specific cancer mortalities show marked geographical preferences, tending to occur together at high, or low, frequency levels, in particular states. It is also clear that some sets of cancer are negatively correlated, mortality from one group being high only in states where that from the other is low and vice versa. A third set of relationships is also apparent; a few cancers do not correlate significantly, either positively or negatively, with any other forms, their distributions appearing to be completely spatially independent. Clearly, cancers with the same spatial distribution may possibly have a common cause. Conversely, strongly negatively correlated groups may be linked through some variable which influences both, but in contrasting directions. Finally, independent distributions suggest a unique cause(s) for the cancer types involved.

The analysis yielded 8,580 Pearson correlation coefficients, which obviously cannot all be described in detail here. However, various highlights should be mentioned. In white males, in the United States, the distribution of esophageal cancer correlates both highly and positively with 10 specific cancers, or groups of cancers, and consequently with that of all malignant neoplasms. The cancers involved are those of the tongue ($r = 0.88582$, $p = 0.0001$), all digestive organs ($r = 0.87948$, $p = 0.0001$), the large intestine [excluding rectum] ($r = 0.87892$, $p = 0.0001$), oral mesopharynx [including tonsils] ($r = 0.86102$, $p = 0.0001$), the rectum ($r = 0.84769$, $p = 0.0001$), and the floor of the mouth ($r = 0.82836$, $p = 0.0001$) (Figure 1,1). Several other cancers also correlate highly with esophageal cancer in white males. These include cancer of the larynx ($r = 0.82791$, $p = 0.0001$) and of the entire buccal cavity and pharynx ($r = 0.82524$, $p = 0.0001$), all urinary tract organs ($r = 0.82132$, $p = 0.0001$) and the bladder and urinary organs ($r = 0.81941$, $p = 0.0001$). As a result of these 10 significant correlations, the spatial distribution of cancer of the esophagus, in white males in the United States, also correlates highly with that for all malignant neoplasms ($r = 0.90687$, $p = 0.0001$). In addition to these apparent relationships, esophageal cancer displays marked positive correlations with cancer of the hypopharynx ($r = 0.69838$, $p = 0.0001$), other parts of the mouth ($r = 0.65451$, $p = 0.0001$), the kidney ($r = 0.64900$, $p = 0.0001$), all respiratory cancer ($r = 0.62854$, $p = 0.0001$), and cancer of the pharynx ($r = 0.61982$, $p = 0.0001$). Even beyond this, its distribution correlates positively, at a moderate level ($r = 0.4$ to 0.6, $p > 0.005$) with seven further cancers, those of the lung, stomach, breast and pancreas and with all lymphomas, Hodgkin's disease and reticulum cell sarcoma.

A similar suite of high, marked and moderate positive correlations was also found to occur in non-white males. In particular, cancer of the floor of the mouth ($r = 0.94063$, $p = 0.0001$), all digestive organs ($r = $

0.90993, p = 0.0001), the entire buccal cavity and pharynx (r = 0.88267, p = 0.0001), oral mesopharynx and tonsils (r = 0.88105, p = 0.0001), tongue (r = 0.85279, p = 0.0001), lung (r = 0.83818, p = 0.0001), all respiratory organs (r = 0.83502, p = 0.0001) and the rectum (r = 0.81947, p = 0.0001) had high positive correlations with esophageal cancer. So too did all malignant neoplasms (r = 0.90539, p = 0.0001). In addition, 10 other specific cancers or cancer groups had marked and 10 had moderate positive correlations with esophageal cancer. Only cancer of the eye (r = −0.40709, p = 0.035) showed any sign of meaningful negative correlation with it (Figure 2,1). While these correlations do not prove a common cause, they strongly suggest some link between many, if not all, cancers of the digestive and respiratory systems in both white and non-white males.

While the strength of correlation tended, overall, to be lower in white females than in white males, certain marked trends were also obvious. Breast cancer, the greatest killer of younger women, correlated both highly and positively with four specific cancers, or cancer groups, namely cancer of the ovary (r = 0.90818, p = 0.0001), of all digestive organs (r = 0.90760, p = 0.0001), the rectum (r = 0.89732, p = 0.0001) and the large intestine (r = 0.88243, p = 0.0001). As a result of these and other relationships, breast cancer in white females also correlated highly with all malignant neoplasms (r = 0.89707, p = 0.0001). In addition, breast cancer displayed a marked degree of positive correlation with six other specific cancers and cancer groups, namely all lymphomas (r = 0.79652, p = 0.0001) and cancer of all urinary tract organs (r = 0.78898, p = 0.0001), Hodgkin's disease (r = 0.70626, p = 0.0001), the small intestine (r = 0.62530, p = 0.0001), the bladder (r = 0.62047, p = 0.0001), and the stomach (r = 0.60056, p = 0.0001). Very interestingly, breast cancer in white females displayed a marked negative correlation with cancer of the skin (r = −0.68164, p = 0.0001), the entire integument (r = −0.66603, p = 0.0001) and melanoma (r = −0.60101, p = 0.0001). The author will suggest, elsewhere in this volume, that these negative correlations may in part reflect an inverse relationship between breast cancer and exposure to sunlight, the significance of which will later become apparent (Figure 3,1).

Breast cancer's spatial distribution also positively correlates to a moderate degree (r = 0.6 to 0.4, p > 0.005) with cancer of the pancreas, peritoneum, uterus, thyroid, reticulum cell sarcoma, genitals, acute leukemia, other reticuloses, kidney and other primary malignant lymphoid neoplasms. Moderate negative correlations were also found with cancer of other parts of the mouth, lip and the entire buccal cavity and pharynx (Figure 1,1).

A similar grouping of high, marked and moderate positive correlations was also found in non-white females (Figure 2,1). In particular, the

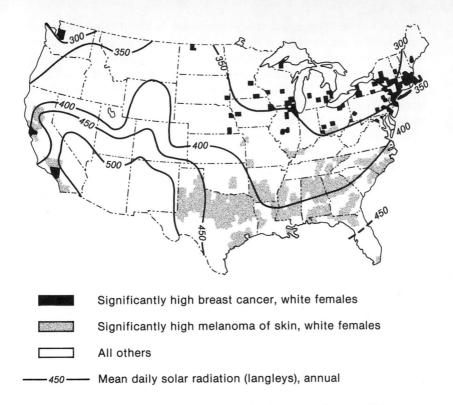

Significantly high breast cancer, white females

Significantly high melanoma of skin, white females

All others

——450—— Mean daily solar radiation (langleys), annual

Figure 3,1 A Comparison of United States Mortality from Breast Cancer and Melanoma in White Females (1950-1969)

distribution of cancer of the large intestine (r = 0.90434, p = 0.0001), ovary (r = 0.85272, p = 0.0001) and rectum (r = 0.82793, p = 0.0001) correlated both highly and positively with the distribution of breast cancer in non-white women. In addition, there were eleven marked positive correlations, namely those between breast cancer and all urinary tract organs, all digestive organs, the pancreas, bladder and urinary tract organs, the nervous system, the tongue, the peritoneum, all lymphomas, the esophagus and reticulum cell sarcoma (Figure 2,1). This group also included all malignant neoplasms (r = 0.74510, p = 0.0001). In non-white women (mainly black females) there was, however, no sign of a negative correlation between breast cancer and cancer of the skin, the entire integument or melanoma. All three of these cancers showed no significant correlation, either negative or positive, with breast cancer.

11

In addition to these major cancer sets, other relationships are apparent from the Pearson correlation matrices. Cancer of the eye, for example, in both white and non-white males, has no high or marked positive correlations with the geographical distribution of any other form of cancer (Figures 1,1 and 2,1). The same is true of cancer of the eye in white women (Figure 1,1). However, its distribution correlates negatively with several cancers in both white men and women, including for males that of the thyroid ($r = -0.53358$, $p = 0.0001$), bladder and urinary tract ($r = -0.46297$, $p = 0.0009$) and all urinary tract organs ($r = -0.45368$, $p = 0.0012$). Even more obviously, negative correlations occur between the spatial distribution of cancer of the eye and other malignant neoplasms in non-white males. For example, cancer of the eye displays moderate negative correlations with nine specific cancers or cancer groups. These are cancer of the nervous system ($r = -0.57227$, $p = 0.0018$), pancreas ($r = -0.51054$, $p = 0.0065$), acute leukemia ($r = -0.49964$, $p = 0.0080$), testes ($r = -0.48792$, $p = 0.0198$), other reticuloses ($r = -0.44834$, $p = 0.0190$), all digestive organs ($r = -0.43769$, $p = 0.0224$), the stomach ($r = -0.40949$, $p = 0.0339$), the esophagus ($r = -0.40709$, $p = 0.0351$) and all urinary tract organs ($r = -0.40002$, $p = 0.0387$). Strangely enough, such negative correlations between cancer of the eye and other malignant neoplasms, in non-white women, occurs at a very much lower level of significance (Figure 2,1).

A lack of high or marked significant correlation also occurs for some types of leukemia, namely myeloid and monocytic. These forms of leukemia show no high, or marked, positive or negative correlations, in white women or white and non-white men, either between themselves or with other cancers. This tends to suggest that both are possibly unique in distribution and cause. In contrast, lymphatic leukemia shows negative correlations with numerous other specific and group cancer distributions in both white men and women, although this trend is more marked in males than in females. To illustrate, in white males lymphatic leukemia correlates negatively with cancer of the larynx ($r = -0.60272$, $p = 0.0001$), tongue ($r = -0.59650$, $p = 0.0001$), all respiratory cancer ($r = -0.58268$, $p = 0.0001$), cancer of the entire buccal cavity ($r = -0.57993$, $p = 0.0001$), lung ($r = -0.56791$, $p = 0.0001$), other parts of the mouth ($r = -0.54840$, $p = 0.0001$), and mycosis fungoides ($r = -0.51269$, $p = 0.0002$). Indeed, lymphatic leukemia correlates negatively at varying levels of significance with 39 out of the possible 55 specific cancers, or groups of cancers, which occur in white males. In white women there are 36 negative correlations out of a possible 61. This type of repeated negative relationship is more pronounced with lymphatic leukemia than with any other cancer type, in either white males or white females.

One final group of relationships also requires comment. This involves marked positive correlations which occur between a group of cancers which include those of the lip, skin, entire integument, bone, other parts of the mouth, the buccal cavity and pharynx, melanoma, the nose and ear and unspecified leukemia. In white females all these cancers correlate with lip cancer with reliable coefficients of correlation > 0.4 and with probabilities > 0.01. Lip cancer and bone cancer, for example, have a marked degree of correlation ($r = 0.68326$, $p = 0.0001$). Interestingly enough, lip cancer correlates moderately negatively in white females with six other cancers, namely those of the breast, ovary, rectum, all urinary tract organs, lymphosarcoma and all lymphomas (Figure 1,1). In non-white females, the only significant moderate negative correlation is with lymphosarcoma ($r = -0.46639$, $p = 0.0142$).

It is clear from the preceding discussion that there are many high and marked positive and negative reliable coefficients of correlation between the distributions of specific cancers in the United States, at the state level. As can be seen from *The Atlas of Cancer Mortality for U.S. Counties: 1950-1969*[13] these correlations stem from links between numerous clusters of high and low death rates for specific cancers, not simply random patterns of cancer deaths.

Factor Analysis

Unfortunately, it is difficult to fully appreciate the relevance of 8,580 correlation coefficients. Magnitude, in and of itself, becomes both an advantage and a disadvantage. What is needed is a technique for summarizing the data without destroying its quality. Factor analysis provides a convenient means of achieving this end. Its purpose is to identify those variables that are closely related to each other, and that are distinct in some way from all the other variables in the same data set.[14]

Factor analyses involve a search for clusters of cancer types which show a high or marked degree of inter-correlation, by computer examination of the Pearson correlation matrices.[15] It determines, therefore, a certain degree of homogeneity among a number of specified variables, that can then be considered subsequently in this new order as a derived variable, that is as a factor.[16] Using this technique the distributions of specific cancer types (groups were omitted) in white and non-white males and females, in the United States, were summarized into a number of new variables or factors. In addition to these four individual factor analyses, the technique was repeated for all of these groups combined. In total, therefore, five factor analyses were undertaken (Figures 5,1 to 9,1).

13

Figure 4,1 Cancer Mortality in the United States (1950-1967):
Factor Analysis Scree Plots of Eigenvalues

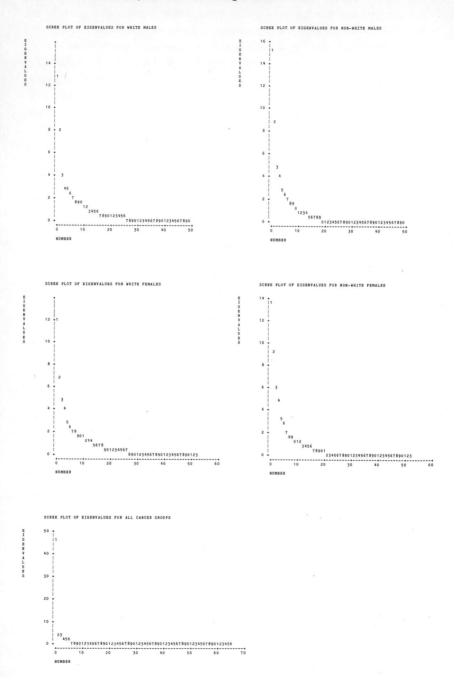

Figure 5,1   White Males: Factor Weighting

FACTOR PATTERN

CANCER TYPE	FACTOR1	FACTOR2	FACTOR3	FACTOR4	FACTOR5	FACTOR6	FACTOR7	FACTOR8	FACTOR9	FACTOR10
TM2M	0.93617	-0.20283	.	.	.	.	.	.	.	.
TM11M	0.92634	.	.	.	.	.	.	.	.	.
TM22M	0.91073	-0.36475	.	.	.	.	.	.	.	.
TM4M	0.90424	.	.	.	.	.	-0.20404	.	.	.
TM14M	0.87760	0.30675	.	.	.	.	.	.	.	.
TM6M	0.87106	.	-0.21180	.	.	.	-0.22509	.	.	.
TM40M	0.86987	0.25621	.	.	.	.	.	.	.	.
TM15M	0.85021	0.43914	.	.	.	.	.	.	.	.
TM5M	0.76651	-0.41857	.	.	.	.	.	.	-0.21474	.
TM8M	0.70044	.	.	.	.	.	-0.42406	.	.	.
TM24M	0.66120	-0.38143	0.27156	-0.26052	.	.	.	-0.34360	.	.
TM9M	0.65170	-0.57643	0.24395	.	.	.	-0.22746	.	.	.
TM50M	0.54928	.	.	0.38620	.	.	.	-0.34909	-0.23761	.
TM53M	0.54038	0.44668	0.36082	.	.	.	.	0.31199	.	.
TM27M	0.49238	0.45561	.	.	.	.	.	0.33268	-0.33688	.
TM54M	0.45616	.	0.23475	0.22647	-0.43423	.	-0.28409	-0.31691	.	.
TM56M	0.45292	-0.22840	-0.38847	.	-0.39785	.	.	.	.	.
TM19M	0.42365	-0.36858	.	.	.	.	0.25758	0.27013	.	.
TM62M	0.41291	.	-0.26832	0.32800	.	.	0.31414	.	.	0.40723
TM59M	-0.49387	0.47696	0.23221	0.26310	0.27058	0.23004	.	.	.	.
TM12M	0.44415	0.69064	.	-0.22071	.	.	.	0.23002	.	.
TM39M	0.61691	0.67144	.	.	.	.	.	.	.	.
TM57M	.	0.61181	.	0.47031	.	.	.	.	.	.
TM35M	.	0.55974	0.38542	0.26061	-0.26604	.	0.21653	.	0.22818	.
TM13M	0.36888	0.42419	.	-0.27333	.	.	.	0.31789	.	.
TM49M	.	0.37075	-0.33529	.	-0.28752	0.26141	-0.24012	.	0.23262	0.33412
TM3M	0.37345	-0.48363	.	0.30101	.	0.21706	0.38713	.	0.27516	.
TM7M	0.32760	-0.62207	.	.	0.34112	.	.	.	.	.
TM65M	0.37880	-0.66378	0.26007	-0.33392	.	.	.	.	.	.
TM2?M	.	-0.81899	.	0.33253	.	.	.	.	.	.
TM43M	-0.24461	-0.81742	.	0.21130	.	.	.	0.29341	.	.
TM63M	.	-0.25791	0.79703	.	.	.	.	.	0.23888	.
TM52M	0.34297	0.29947	0.52439	0.32470	.	.	.	.	.	.
TM55M	0.33136	0.38541	0.49823	0.25906	.	.	-0.20914	.	.	.
TM48M	0.40862	-0.36394	0.44452	-0.22701	.	0.26311	0.32759	0.27684	.	.
TM23M	0.31790	-0.36618	-0.46426	0.40085	.	0.21832	.	0.23540	.	.
TM16M	0.31350	.	-0.50669	.	0.27926	.	.	0.34154	0.21307	.
TM47M	.	0.40488	-0.54104	.	.	.	.	.	.	-0.33683
TM51M	.	.	-0.63363	.	0.35588	0.44144	.	.	.	.
TM46M	.	.	.	0.68065	0.24205	0.40988	.	0.22528	.	.
TM17M	0.50748	.	.	0.51551	0.25544	.	.	.	.	0.23770
TM60M	.	0.28179	.	.	0.55918	-0.46625	0.20690	.	.	0.43399
TM45M	-0.32497	-0.31229	0.20382	0.23422	0.50823	.	-0.25327	.	.	-0.20192
TM25M	0.25051	-0.32014	.	-0.34307	0.50009	.	.	.	.	.
TM37M	0.28128	.	0.24011	.	-0.31182	0.61288	0.38115	.	.	.
TM1M	-0.29232	.	0.23428	-0.21473	.	0.46588	.	0.22377	.	.
TM36M	.	0.36006	.	.	0.40506	0.45936	0.24437	-0.40480	0.20800	.
TM18M	0.31286	0.32240	0.24194	.	0.23869	.	0.38197	-0.24376	-0.27700	-0.35512
TM21M	.	.	.	.	-0.34762	-0.34961	.	.	0.69853	-0.20201
TM61M	.	-0.25974	.	.	0.22744	0.37543	-0.27869	-0.22327	0.31839	-0.55462

NOTE: VALUES LESS THAN 0.2 HAVE BEEN SHOWN AS '.'

EIGENVALUES OF THE CORRELATION MATRIX: TOTAL = 50.000000   AVERAGE = 1.000000

	1	2	3	4	5	6	7	8	9
EIGENVALUE	12.717600	7.919820	3.945894	2.910450	2.655486	2.336099	1.868039	1.734159	1.614946
DIFFERENCE	4.797780	3.973926	1.035444	0.254964	0.319388	0.468060	0.133880	0.119213	0.092214
PROPORTION	0.2544	0.1584	0.0789	0.0582	0.0531	0.0467	0.0374	0.0347	0.0323
CUMULATIVE	0.2544	0.4127	0.4917	0.5499	0.6030	0.6497	0.6871	0.7218	0.7540

	10	11	12	13	14	15	16	17	18
EIGENVALUE	1.522732	1.292723	1.161493	0.965400	0.832050	0.795268	0.689270	0.590010	0.504505
DIFFERENCE	0.230010	0.131230	0.196094	0.133349	0.036782	0.105999	0.099260	0.085505	0.020685
PROPORTION	0.0305	0.0259	0.0232	0.0193	0.0166	0.0159	0.0138	0.0118	0.0101
CUMULATIVE	0.7845	0.8104	0.8336	0.8529	0.8695	0.8854	0.8992	0.9110	0.9211

	19	20	21	22	23	24	25	26	27
EIGENVALUE	0.483821	0.437706	0.416251	0.378730	0.348190	0.331357	0.270747	0.240256	0.156256
DIFFERENCE	0.046115	0.021454	0.037521	0.030540	0.016834	0.060610	0.030491	0.084000	0.011777
PROPORTION	0.0097	0.0088	0.0083	0.0076	0.0070	0.0066	0.0054	0.0048	0.0031
CUMULATIVE	0.9308	0.9395	0.9479	0.9554	0.9624	0.9690	0.9745	0.9793	0.9824

	28	29	30	31	32	33	34	35	36
EIGENVALUE	0.144479	0.131808	0.110199	0.100924	0.069022	0.056877	0.052637	0.044224	0.043030
DIFFERENCE	0.012671	0.021609	0.009275	0.031903	0.012144	0.004240	0.008413	0.001194	0.014307
PROPORTION	0.0029	0.0026	0.0022	0.0020	0.0014	0.0011	0.0011	0.0009	0.0009
CUMULATIVE	0.9853	0.9879	0.9901	0.9921	0.9935	0.9947	0.9957	0.9966	0.9974

	37	38	39	40	41	42	43	44	45
EIGENVALUE	0.028723	0.025962	0.023668	0.018333	0.009341	0.009050	0.004963	0.003831	0.002384
DIFFERENCE	0.002761	0.002294	0.005334	0.008993	0.000291	0.004087	0.001132	0.001447	0.001475
PROPORTION	0.0006	0.0005	0.0005	0.0004	0.0002	0.0002	0.0001	0.0001	0.0000
CUMULATIVE	0.9980	0.9985	0.9990	0.9994	0.9996	0.9998	0.9999	0.9999	1.0000

	46	47	48	49	50
EIGENVALUE	0.000909	0.000380	0.000000	0.000000	-0.000000
DIFFERENCE	0.000529	0.000380	0.000000	0.000000	
PROPORTION	0.0000	0.0000	0.0000	0.0000	-0.0000
CUMULATIVE	1.0000	1.0000	1.0000	1.0000	1.0000

FINAL COMMUNALITY ESTIMATES: TOTAL = 39.225227

TM1M	TM2M	TM3M	TM4M	TM5M	TM6M	TM7M	TM8M	TM9M	TM11M
0.567223	0.950603	0.764560	0.901968	0.891138	0.937048	0.715306	0.750687	0.884878	0.908362

TM12M	TM13M	TM14M	TM15M	TM16M	TM17M	TM18M	TM19M	TM21M	TM22M
0.842600	0.544265	0.910820	0.933127	0.680682	0.766136	0.756067	0.601387	0.806417	0.968917

TM23M	TM24M	TM25M	TM27M	TM35M	TM36M	TM37M	TM39M	TM40M	TM42M
0.754341	0.878895	0.619230	0.768157	0.728373	0.799871	0.803763	0.900395	0.892340	0.839416

TM43M	TM45M	TM46M	TM47M	TM48M	TM49M	TM50M	TM51M	TM52M	TM53M
0.923518	0.856129	0.798653	0.703417	0.831842	0.664565	0.737177	0.838025	0.648706	0.757081

TM54M	TM55M	TM56M	TM57M	TM59M	TM60M	TM61M	TM62M	TM63M	TM65M
0.741797	0.663323	0.613977	0.710536	0.805762	0.769725	0.825312	0.646322	0.813563	0.837665

See page 3 for key.

15

Figure 6,1   Non-White Males: Factor Weighting

```
KEY:    FACTOR1   DIGESTIVE-MULTIPLE MYELOMA              FACTOR6    GENITAL-PHARYNX
        FACTOR2   GENITAL-LIP                             FACTOR7    LYMPHATIC LEUKEMIA-LYMPHOID NEOPLASMS
        FACTOR3   BONE-PERITONEUM                         FACTOR8    EYE-BONE
        FACTOR4   MYCOSIS FUNGOIDES-DIGESTIVE             FACTOR9    PROSTATE-OTHER RETICULOSES
        FACTOR5   BONE-BREAST                             FACTOR10   SKIN-GENITALS
```

FACTOR PATTERN

CANCER TYPE	FACTOR1	FACTOR2	FACTOR3	FACTOR4	FACTOR5	FACTOR6	FACTOR7	FACTOR8	FACTOR9	FACTOR10
TM15NWM	0.92533	.	.	.	.	-0.20316	.	.	.	.
TM11NWM	0.88928	.	0.28836	.	.	.	.	.	.	.
TM57NWM	0.88585	.	.	-0.26255	.	.	.	.	0.21472	.
TM4NWM	0.88471	.	.	.	.	.	.	.	-0.22880	.
TM14NWM	0.86833	.	.	.	.	.	0.23638	.	.	.
TM8NWM	0.86392	.	.	0.22764	-0.23161	.	.	.	.	.
TM24NWM	0.85994	.	0.26715	.	.	.	.	.	0.23620	.
TM17NWM	0.84700	0.23581	.	-0.22390	.	.	.	.	.	.
TM2NWM	0.82233	.	0.26771	.	0.20873	.	.	.	-0.20405	.
TM22NWM	0.80301	-0.34958	.	.	0.24743	.	0.20868	.	.	.
TM6NWM	0.79953	.	0.39823	-0.27117	.	.	-0.21777	.	.	.
TM40NWM	0.78061	0.21776	.	.	.	.	-0.44638	.	.	.
TM50NWM	0.72554	.	-0.32633	.	-0.24350	.	0.34064	.	.	.
TM23NWM	0.71354	.	-0.27579	.	0.36137	-0.30371	.	.	.	.
TM51NWM	0.67736	.	-0.57933	.	.	.	.	.	.	.
TM12NWM	0.66694	0.20493	0.37202	.	.	.	.	.	.	-0.27199
TM5NWM	0.62305	-0.31433	.	0.44158	-0.21102	.	0.32772	.	.	.
TM49NWM	0.61159	-0.49216	-0.46741	.	.	.	.	.	.	.
TM13NWM	0.58973	-0.33119	-0.28848	0.33031	0.24030	.	.	0.25197	.	.
TM53NWM	0.56820	.	0.38072	-0.55311	.	0.25595	.	.	.	.
TM7NWM	0.54946	.	-0.54337	0.29239	-0.33743	.	.	.	-0.32533	.
TM59NWM	0.44574	.	-0.39674	-0.36851	.	0.20942	0.39727	0.25221	0.23956	.
TM3NWM	0.43835	-0.39484	.	.	-0.24784	0.36901	-0.29979	0.37855	-0.34146	.
TM39NWM	0.27275	0.88401	.	.	.	.	.	.	.	.
TM36NWM	.	0.87923	0.21634	.	0.22350	.	.	.	.	.
TM1NWM	.	0.83843	.	.	0.34592	0.26510	.	.	.	.
TM46NWM	0.31933	0.81494	.	.	0.34576	.	.	.	.	.
TM62NWM	0.21884	0.77074	.	.	.	.	0.23932	.	-0.25124	0.25375
TM21NWM	.	0.72011	0.52332	.	.	-0.30304	.	.	.	.
TM47NWM	0.34956	0.69728	.	.	.	.	-0.32399	.	.	.
TM63NWM	-0.24955	0.60138	.	0.47407	.	0.26043	.	.	.	.
TM16NWM	0.40392	0.56585	.	.	-0.32156	-0.30185	.	.	-0.31955	.
TM55NWM	0.42275	0.50019	-0.25281	-0.36156	.	.	-0.25960	-0.26650	0.40196	.
TM60NWM	0.27839	-0.55664	.	-0.43517	0.23298	.	0.31153	.	-0.22090	.
TM27NWM	.	-0.61140	.	.	0.46146	-0.23098	.	.	.	.
TM35NWM	0.50572	-0.63119	.	-0.26697	.	.	.	.	0.42162	.
TM65NWM	.	0.30206	0.67800	.	.	.	0.24015	.	.	-0.20646
TM4NWM	.	.	0.51204	0.35812	0.40262	.	.	0.40611	0.25801	.
TM18NWM	0.30455	-0.42706	0.50049	.	.	-0.24919	-0.46912	.	.	.
TM43NWM	.	-0.45562	0.48117	0.29999	0.39833	-0.25189	.	.	.	0.31164
TM54NWM	0.26036	.	-0.72775	0.43386	.	0.27129	.	.	0.23177	.
TM56NWM	0.52199	.	.	0.56590	.	-0.28788	.	.	.	.
TM61NWM	0.23592	0.39227	0.22108	-0.50921	.	-0.36592	.	0.39806	.	.
TM52NWM	0.42141	-0.25394	.	-0.57453	-0.27201	.	0.34312	-0.21577	.	.
TM25NWM	0.21283	-0.34034	.	0.45896	-0.56325	-0.30506	.	.	.	0.26818
TM42NWM	0.28309	.	0.47653	.	-0.64193	0.21809	.	.	0.22840	0.22874
TM37NWM	-0.22391	-0.24670	.	0.25872	0.31224	0.58313	.	-0.30798	.	0.32221
TM9NWM	0.46259	-0.31873	0.31817	.	.	0.57039	0.20542	.	.	.
TM45NWM	-0.35234	-0.40469	.	0.22161	-0.33635	.	.	.	0.60949	-0.20507
TM19NWM	.	.	0.43563	0.54962	.	.	.	.	.	-0.58032

NOTE: VALUES LESS THAN 0.2 HAVE BEEN SHOWN AS '.'

EIGENVALUES OF THE CORRELATION MATRIX: TOTAL = 50.000000   AVERAGE = 1.000000

	1	2	3	4	5	6	7	8	9
EIGENVALUE	15.180121	8.783872	4.923084	3.998153	2.866898	2.373629	2.074662	1.588507	1.522421
DIFFERENCE	6.396249	3.860788	0.924931	1.131254	0.493269	0.298967	0.486155	0.066086	0.319018
PROPORTION	0.3036	0.1757	0.0985	0.0800	0.0573	0.0475	0.0415	0.0318	0.0304
CUMULATIVE	0.3036	0.4793	0.5777	0.6577	0.7150	0.7625	0.8040	0.8358	0.8662

	10	11	12	13	14	15	16	17	18
EIGENVALUE	1.203403	0.867142	0.763802	0.658868	0.619513	0.459623	0.419779	0.363804	0.319787
DIFFERENCE	0.336261	0.103340	0.104934	0.039355	0.159890	0.039844	0.055975	0.044017	0.050624
PROPORTION	0.0241	0.0173	0.0153	0.0132	0.0124	0.0092	0.0084	0.0073	0.0064
CUMULATIVE	0.8903	0.9076	0.9229	0.9361	0.9485	0.9577	0.9661	0.9733	0.9797

	19	20	21	22	23	24	25	26	27
EIGENVALUE	0.269164	0.178465	0.159033	0.128997	0.090802	0.082399	0.062441	0.041632	0.000000
DIFFERENCE	0.090699	0.019432	0.030036	0.038195	0.008404	0.019958	0.020809	0.041632	0.000000
PROPORTION	0.0054	0.0036	0.0032	0.0026	0.0018	0.0016	0.0012	0.0008	0.0000
CUMULATIVE	0.9851	0.9887	0.9919	0.9945	0.9963	0.9979	0.9992	1.0000	1.0000

	28	29	30	31	32	33	34	35	36
EIGENVALUE	0.000000	0.000000	0.000000	0.000000	0.000000	0.000000	0.000000	0.000000	0.000000
DIFFERENCE	0.000000	0.000000	0.000000	0.000000	0.000000	0.000000	0.000000	0.000000	0.000000
PROPORTION	0.0000	0.0000	0.0000	0.0000	0.0000	0.0000	0.0000	0.0000	0.0000
CUMULATIVE	1.0000	1.0000	1.0000	1.0000	1.0000	1.0000	1.0000	1.0000	1.0000

	37	38	39	40	41	42	43	44	45
EIGENVALUE	0.000000	0.000000	0.000000	0.000000	0.000000	0.000000	0.000000	0.000000	0.000000
DIFFERENCE	0.000000	0.000000	0.000000	0.000000	0.000000	0.000000	0.000000	0.000000	0.000000
PROPORTION	0.0000	0.0000	0.0000	0.0000	0.0000	0.0000	0.0000	0.0000	0.0000
CUMULATIVE	1.0000	1.0000	1.0000	1.0000	1.0000	1.0000	1.0000	1.0000	1.0000

	46	47	48	49	50
EIGENVALUE	0.000000	0.000000	0.000000	-0.000000	-0.000000
DIFFERENCE	0.000000	0.000000	0.000000	0.000000	
PROPORTION	0.0000	0.0000	0.0000	-0.0000	-0.0000
CUMULATIVE	1.0000	1.0000	1.0000	1.0000	1.0000

FINAL COMMUNALITY ESTIMATES: TOTAL = 44.514749

TM1NWM	TM2NWM	TM3NWM	TM4NWM	TM5NWM	TM6NWM	TM7NWM	TM8NWM	TM9NWM	TM11NWM
0.956929	0.889981	0.922719	0.946169	0.865945	0.976779	0.931437	0.921732	0.851834	0.924847

TM12NWM	TM13NWM	TM14NWM	TM15NWM	TM16NWM	TM17NWM	TM18NWM	TM19NWM	TM21NWM	TM22NWM
0.780564	0.873263	0.902306	0.953413	0.883663	0.909182	0.850772	0.884388	0.907559	0.942750

TM23NWM	TM24NWM	TM25NWM	TM27NWM	TM35NWM	TM36NWM	TM37NWM	TM39NWM	TM40NWM	TM42NWM
0.889144	0.955003	0.907073	0.758894	0.955359	0.953483	0.842869	0.943128	0.915052	0.888297

TM43NWM	TM45NWM	TM46NWM	TM47NWM	TM48NWM	TM49NWM	TM50NWM	TM51NWM	TM52NWM	TM53NWM
0.905840	0.911957	0.939475	0.862088	0.832381	0.901118	0.880664	0.913761	0.817890	0.895015

TM54NWM	TM55NWM	TM56NWM	TM57NWM	TM59NWM	TM60NWM	TM61NWM	TM62NWM	TM63NWM	TM65NWM
0.952496	0.941480	0.777009	0.950607	0.856766	0.807460	0.851133	0.894649	0.781565	0.756860

See page 3 for key.

16

Figure 7,1 White Females: Factor Weighting

KEY:
FACTOR1 GENITAL-DIGESTIVE
FACTOR2 RESPIRATORY-DIGESTIVE
FACTOR3 RESPIRATORY
FACTOR4 NERVOUS SYSTEM-MULTIPLE MYELOMA
FACTOR5 MEDIASTINUM-GIANT FOLLICULAR
        LYMPHOMA

FACTOR6 NOSE-THYROID
FACTOR7 MONOCYTIC LEUKEMIA
FACTOR8 UTERUS-GENITAL
FACTOR9 LIVER-UTERUS
FACTOR10 MONOCYTIC LEUKEMIA-LYMPHOID
         NEOPLASMS

FACTOR PATTERN

CANCER TYPE	FACTOR1	FACTOR2	FACTOR3	FACTOR4	FACTOR5	FACTOR6	FACTOR7	FACTOR8	FACTOR9	FACTOR10
TM32F	0.89943	.	.	.	.	.	.	.	.	.
TM27F	0.89531	0.31349	.	.	.	.	.	.	.	.
TM15F	0.79153	0.50694	.	.	.	.	.	.	.	.
TM13F	0.75012	.	-0.29298	0.20598	.	-0.22357	.	.	.	.
TM14F	0.74306	0.48312	-0.22759	.	.	.	.	.	.	.
TM53F	0.72606	.	-0.21916	0.25031	0.24402	0.20834	.	.	.	.
TM12F	0.66501	.	-0.37089	.	.	.	-0.38532	.	.	.
TM39F	0.64631	-0.28716	-0.36157	.	.	.	.	.	.	-0.26910
TM16F	0.63768	-0.40880	.	.	-0.31785	.	.	.	0.27351	.
TM47F	0.59859	-0.23574	.	.	.	0.55381	.	.	.	.
TM17F	0.58018	0.41190	.	0.21467	.	.	.	.	.	-0.35917
TM29F	0.57711	.	0.29410	0.26026	.	.	.	0.22427	0.21511	.
TM18F	0.53108	.	.	.	.	0.41221	.	.	.	0.31410
TM49F	0.50914	.	0.34548	.	0.26014	.	.	-0.33021	-0.35694	.
TM50F	0.45509	0.39418	0.31227	0.25526	-0.33956	-0.32776	.	.	.	.
TM52F	0.42544	.	.	0.41894	0.25594	-0.27592	.	-0.25578	.	0.32857
TM51F	0.41485	-0.35064	0.28372	-0.30474	.	0.38601	.	.	.	-0.21521
TM9F	-0.56622	0.40140	.	0.23961	0.32554	.	.	.	0.22063	.
TM1F	-0.61737	.	.	0.45868	.	.	.	-0.28181	.	.
TM42F	-0.71107	.	0.20452	0.39684	.	.	.	.	-0.34996	.
TM5F	-0.75357	0.29980	.	0.35144	.	.	.	.	.	.
TM43F	-0.83821	.	.	0.34795	.	.	.	.	.	.
TM40F	0.37108	0.81341	.	.	.	.	.	.	.	.
TM11F	.	0.80173	.	0.41550	.	.	.	.	.	.
TM22F	-0.26830	0.72543	.	.	-0.21590	.	.	0.24743	.	.
TM24F	.	0.64243	.	-0.43442	0.29288	.	.	.	-0.30389	.
TM6F	.	0.53008	0.41546	-0.24297	0.21633	.	.	-0.30515	.	.
TM28F	-0.51899	0.52285	.	.	.	.	0.39964	.	.	.
TM65F	-0.30218	0.50592	-0.34252	-0.41244	.	0.22997	.	.	.	.
TM19F	-0.21415	0.50432	.	.	.	.	-0.34638	.	.	.
TM8F	.	0.48239	0.29451	.	0.24609	-0.35785	0.21236	0.33796	-0.23226	.
TM3F	-0.37106	-0.39147	.	0.23086	.	.	.	.	.	-0.22557
TM59F	.	-0.56526	.	0.24482	.	.	0.29403	.	.	.
TM4F	.	0.33322	0.60266	0.33408	.	.	.	.	0.20401	0.27864
TM23F	.	.	0.57770	0.27093	-0.27788	.	.	-0.38422	0.24610	.
TM2F	-0.23421	0.32584	0.54294	.	-0.21292	0.31226	.	.	.	0.23371
TM56F	.	0.28250	0.37340	-0.34131	-0.33288	.	.	.	.	-0.20629
TM53F	0.38261	0.35053	-0.40005	.	-0.26528	.	0.30871	0.38498	.	.
TM55F	0.41858	.	-0.44481	0.32777	0.25433	-0.26508	.	.	.	.
TM46F	-0.47114	0.22600	-0.47635	0.35477	-0.21244	0.41106	.	.	.	.
TM31F	.	0.39140	-0.55358	-0.28080	-0.23089	.	0.32936	.	.	.
TM63F	-0.39840	.	-0.60085	0.22430	.	.	.	.	-0.27325	.
TM46F	.	.	0.31705	0.60221	-0.28132	.	.	0.24245	0.21671	.
TM57F	0.42069	.	.	0.56953	0.31370	.	.	.	-0.31827	.
TM54F	.	.	.	0.34183	0.71629	.	.	.	.	.
TM25F	.	.	.	-0.34343	0.64742	0.26495	.	.	.	.
TM21F	-0.27777	.	.	0.28578	.	0.62790	.	-0.22256	.	.
TM61F	.	.	.	.	.	.	0.66589	-0.23419	-0.24586	0.45880
TM60F	0.28922	-0.22016	.	0.20411	-0.32953	.	-0.38335	0.33084	-0.22366	.
TM62F	0.38080	0.28303	0.37056	.	.	.	-0.53852	.	.	.
TM30F	.	-0.35812	0.34840	-0.20344	0.22615	.	.	0.44161	0.25389	0.29963
TM7F	.	0.33000	0.42982	.	.	.	.	-0.52983	.	-0.34567
TM45F	-0.20682	-0.33117	0.30461	0.30262	0.24278	.	.	.	0.46627	.

NOTE: VALUES LESS THAN 0.2 HAVE BEEN SHOWN AS '.'

EIGENVALUES OF THE CORRELATION MATRIX: TOTAL = 53.000000   AVERAGE = 1.000000

	1	2	3	4	5	6	7	8	9
EIGENVALUE	11.940098	6.955624	4.627590	3.999313	2.917022	2.433348	2.063170	1.988594	1.732529
DIFFERENCE	4.984474	2.328034	0.628276	1.082292	0.483673	0.370178	0.074576	0.256065	0.210985
PROPORTION	0.2253	0.1312	0.0873	0.0755	0.0550	0.0459	0.0389	0.0375	0.0327
CUMULATIVE	0.2253	0.3565	0.4438	0.5193	0.5743	0.6202	0.6592	0.6967	0.7294

	10	11	12	13	14	15	16	17	18
EIGENVALUE	1.521544	1.415467	1.369456	1.128290	1.099480	0.923687	0.824092	0.678209	0.649959
DIFFERENCE	0.106077	0.046011	0.240158	0.069818	0.135593	0.099795	0.145883	0.028250	0.080285
PROPORTION	0.0287	0.0267	0.0258	0.0213	0.0200	0.0174	0.0155	0.0128	0.0123
CUMULATIVE	0.7581	0.7848	0.8106	0.8319	0.8519	0.8694	0.8849	0.8977	0.9100

	19	20	21	22	23	24	25	26	27
EIGENVALUE	0.569674	0.535069	0.465588	0.423157	0.378001	0.331840	0.265422	0.248494	0.231371
DIFFERENCE	0.034605	0.069481	0.042432	0.045156	0.046161	0.066418	0.016928	0.015123	0.032213
PROPORTION	0.0107	0.0101	0.0088	0.0080	0.0071	0.0063	0.0050	0.0047	0.0044
CUMULATIVE	0.9207	0.9308	0.9396	0.9476	0.9547	0.9610	0.9660	0.9706	0.9750

	28	29	30	31	32	33	34	35	36
EIGENVALUE	0.199158	0.185255	0.169161	0.137833	0.118538	0.088075	0.073660	0.059220	0.054905
DIFFERENCE	0.013903	0.016094	0.031328	0.019295	0.030463	0.014415	0.014440	0.004315	0.001696
PROPORTION	0.0038	0.0035	0.0032	0.0026	0.0022	0.0017	0.0014	0.0011	0.0010
CUMULATIVE	0.9788	0.9823	0.9855	0.9881	0.9903	0.9919	0.9933	0.9945	0.9955

	37	38	39	40	41	42	43	44	45
EIGENVALUE	0.053208	0.047853	0.034502	0.029485	0.025555	0.020630	0.014841	0.006287	0.004663
DIFFERENCE	0.005355	0.013351	0.005018	0.003930	0.004925	0.005788	0.008554	0.001618	0.003609
PROPORTION	0.0010	0.0009	0.0007	0.0006	0.0005	0.0004	0.0003	0.0001	0.0001
CUMULATIVE	0.9965	0.9974	0.9981	0.9986	0.9991	0.9995	0.9998	0.9999	1.0000

	46	47	48	49	50	51	52	53	
EIGENVALUE	0.001060	0.000808	0.000000	0.000000	0.000000	0.000000	0.000000	-0.000000	
DIFFERENCE	0.000252	0.000808	0.000000	0.000000	0.000000	0.000000	0.000000		
PROPORTION	0.0000	0.0000	0.0000	0.0000	0.0000	0.0000	0.0000	-0.0000	
CUMULATIVE	1.0000	1.0000	1.0000	1.0000	1.0000	1.0000	1.0000	1.0000	

FINAL COMMUNALITY ESTIMATES: TOTAL = 40.178833

TM1F	TM2F	TM3F	TM4F	TM5F	TM6F	TM7F	TM8F	TM9F	TM11F	TM12F
0.812476	0.620910	0.499346	0.755753	0.831033	0.685117	0.759068	0.672095	0.763090	0.881877	0.829254

TM13F	TM14F	TM15F	TM16F	TM17F	TM18F	TM19F	TM21F	TM22F	TM23F	TM24F
0.876679	0.906474	0.940944	0.790020	0.750465	0.682908	0.527835	0.670105	0.710070		0.710070

TM25F	TM27F	TM28F	TM29F	TM30F	TM31F	TM32F	TM33F	TM39F	TM40F	TM42F
0.720912	0.931941	0.815468	0.624439	0.734885	0.770061	0.864729	0.839463	0.784743	0.867733	0.896921

TM43F	TM45F	TM46F	TM47F	TM48F	TM49F	TM50F	TM51F	TM52F	TM53F	TM54F
0.901583	0.672482	0.745501	0.781776	0.854195	0.791572	0.800632	0.754817	0.728222	0.812209	0.760641

TM55F	TM56F	TM57F	TM59F	TM60F	TM61F	TM62F	TM63F	TM65F		
0.671679	0.558429	0.755511	0.530235	0.621056	0.849802	0.732774	0.676675	0.778947		

See page 3 for key.

17

Figure 8,1 Non-White Females: Factor Weighting

KEY:
FACTOR1	BREAST-DIGESTIVE	FACTOR6	STOMACH-LIP
FACTOR2	LIVER-THYROID	FACTOR7	MOUTH-GENITAL
FACTOR3	SALIVARY GLAND-MOUTH	FACTOR8	DIGESTIVE-MONOCYTIC LEUKEMIA
FACTOR4	HYPOPHARYNX-CONNECTIVE TISSUE	FACTOR9	MYCOSIS FUNGOIDES
FACTOR5	LYMPHOSARCOMA-STOMACH	FACTOR10	NOSE

FACTOR PATTERN

CANCER TYPE	FACTOR1	FACTOR2	FACTOR3	FACTOR4	FACTOR5	FACTOR6	FACTOR7	FACTOR8	FACTOR9	FACTOR10
TM27NWF	0.85546	.	0.26808	0.21827	.	.	.	.	.	.
TM50NWF	0.84400	.	.	.	.	.	.	.	.	.
TM46NWF	0.83492	.	0.24166	.	.	.	.	.	.	.
TM2NWF	0.82903	.	.	.	.	0.21005	.	.	.	.
TM18NWF	0.81699	.	-0.21531	.	-0.35711	.	.	.	.	.
TM14NWF	0.81046	0.31240	0.29531	.	.	.	.	.	.	.
TM11NWF	0.80482	.	-0.22806	.	.	.	0.33699	.	.	-0.21923
TM32NWF	0.77402	0.39496	0.22248	0.29822	.	.	.	.	.	.
TM15NWF	0.75119	.	0.56122	.	.	.	.	.	.	.
TM29NWF	0.71544	.	-0.48047	0.22451	0.22055	.	.	.	.	.
TM17NWF	0.71505	0.58935	.	.	.	.	.	.	.	.
TM40NWF	0.71023	.	.	0.30106	-0.30235	0.29188	.	.	.	.
TM62NWF	0.66450	.	.	-0.20412	.	.	-0.47182	.	.	.
TM6NWF	0.63702	.	.	-0.58137	-0.28704	.	.	.	.	.
TM60NWF	0.62433	-0.26283	-0.50587	.	.	.	.	.	.	.
TM53NWF	0.60764	0.46792	.	.	.	-0.21865	0.20736	.	-0.21075	.
TM55NWF	0.60296	.	.	-0.25217	.	.	.	0.33988	.	0.27931
TM59NWF	0.54460	-0.47539	.	0.28036	.	0.36590	.	.	.	.
TM61NWF	0.48772	.	.	.	.	.	.	0.39449	-0.39793	0.22274
TM28NWF	-0.41428	0.38030	-0.39764	0.32349	.	-0.40765	.	.	0.23676	.
TM31NWF	-0.52731	-0.44728	.	.	-0.31366	.	.	.	.	.
TM63NWF	-0.53557	.	.	.	0.41147	0.34094	0.26271	0.21815	0.20366	.
TM65NWF	-0.60934	0.43216	.	.	-0.20127	0.22299	0.31501	.	-0.25782	.
TM16NWF	-0.29960	0.91609	.	.	.	.	.	.	.	.
TM47NWF	.	0.85543	.	.	-0.28705	.	.	.	.	.
TM24NWF	.	0.83735	0.24212	.	.	.	.	.	.	.
TM39NWF	.	0.80745	0.40204	.	0.24029	.	.	.	.	.
TM52NWF	-0.25967	0.73974	.	0.31345	0.25702	.	-0.25856	.	.	.
TM21NWF	.	0.70873	.	.	.	0.39803	.	.	.	0.39057
TM57NWF	0.36762	0.68509	0.48092	.	.	.	.	.	.	.
TM23NWF	0.28017	0.58630	.	0.57302	.	.	-0.29712	.	.	.
TM19NWF	-0.28379	0.52838	.	.	.	0.40042	.	0.38109	0.22413	.
TM43NWF	0.29529	-0.57334	-0.21418	-0.40332	.	.	.	.	.	.
TM9NWF	-0.24960	-0.59222	0.36945	.	0.38082	.	0.28824	.	.	.
TM48NWF	.	-0.70548	.	0.30358	0.20364	0.25358	.	-0.25149	.	.
TM3NWF	.	-0.27595	0.68186	.	0.35220	-0.23870	.	0.26471	.	.
TM4NWF	0.26839	.	0.61223	0.28577	.	-0.32830	0.41373	.	.	.
TM25NWF	.	.	0.57101	-0.30837	0.35409	.	.	0.30141	.	0.21244
TM30NWF	0.23066	-0.25986	-0.41834	.	.	-0.33455	.	.	-0.24136	.
TM5NWF	0.40183	.	-0.58335	-0.41114	.	.	0.31252	0.33558	.	.
TM7NWF	0.49021	.	-0.59465	.	0.31659	.	.	.	.	.
TM13NWF	0.63807	.	-0.65267	-0.20591	.	.	.	.	.	.
TM45NWF	0.26547	.	-0.83222	0.20253	0.30256	.	.	.	.	.
TM8NWF	0.30453	.	.	0.65737	-0.44103	.	.	.	.	0.26717
TM49NWF	0.42315	-0.30126	.	0.64581	-0.23992	-0.22432	.	.	.	.
TM33NWF	.	.	-0.21648	0.57685	.	-0.41185	0.40758	.	0.31573	0.25554
TM1NWF	.	-0.31476	.	0.56308	-0.31963	0.44506	.	.	0.21435	.
TM42NWF	0.33339	-0.39340	0.40772	-0.46481	-0.28972	.	-0.23564	.	0.30415	.
TM56NWF	0.38076	.	.	-0.63829	-0.43844	.	.	.	0.32390	.
TM51NWF	0.31452	0.33833	0.37823	.	0.69435	.	.	-0.23795	.	.
TM12NWF	.	0.28673	.	0.28208	0.50582	0.48097	.	.	0.30878	.
TM22NWF	.	0.32883	0.49694	.	.	-0.52592	.	0.35725	0.28672	-0.22870
TM54NWF	.	.	.	0.39795	-0.21435	-0.34743	-0.22801	0.34821	-0.28481	-0.45738

NOTE: VALUES LESS THAN 0.2 HAVE BEEN SHOWN AS '.'

EIGENVALUES OF THE CORRELATION MATRIX: TOTAL = 53.000000 AVERAGE = 1.000000

	1	2	3	4	5	6	7	8	9
EIGENVALUE	13.476599	9.041504	6.107308	4.726478	3.305454	2.745640	1.849284	1.504857	1.438028
DIFFERENCE	4.435096	2.934195	1.380831	1.421024	0.559813	0.896356	0.344427	0.066829	0.131811
PROPORTION	0.2543	0.1706	0.1152	0.0892	0.0624	0.0518	0.0349	0.0284	0.0271
CUMULATIVE	0.2543	0.4249	0.5401	0.6293	0.6916	0.7435	0.7783	0.8067	0.8339

	10	11	12	13	14	15	16	17	18
EIGENVALUE	1.306217	1.227397	1.031789	0.869553	0.686575	0.653958	0.602408	0.471973	0.418345
DIFFERENCE	0.078821	0.195608	0.162235	0.182979	0.032616	0.051550	0.130435	0.053628	0.049310
PROPORTION	0.0246	0.0232	0.0195	0.0164	0.0130	0.0123	0.0114	0.0089	0.0079
CUMULATIVE	0.8585	0.8817	0.9011	0.9175	0.9305	0.9428	0.9542	0.9631	0.9710

	19	20	21	22	23	24	25	26	27
EIGENVALUE	0.369035	0.343559	0.253595	0.191784	0.135856	0.108124	0.096236	0.038442	0.000000
DIFFERENCE	0.025476	0.089965	0.061810	0.055928	0.027732	0.011888	0.057795	0.038442	0.000000
PROPORTION	0.0070	0.0065	0.0048	0.0036	0.0026	0.0020	0.0018	0.0007	0.0000
CUMULATIVE	0.9780	0.9845	0.9892	0.9929	0.9954	0.9975	0.9993	1.0000	1.0000

	28	29	30	31	32	33	34	35	36
EIGENVALUE	0.000000	0.000000	0.000000	0.000000	0.000000	0.000000	0.000000	0.000000	0.000000
DIFFERENCE	0.000000	0.000000	0.000000	0.000000	0.000000	0.000000	0.000000	0.000000	0.000000
PROPORTION	0.0000	0.0000	0.0000	0.0000	0.0000	0.0000	0.0000	0.0000	0.0000
CUMULATIVE	1.0000	1.0000	1.0000	1.0000	1.0000	1.0000	1.0000	1.0000	1.0000

	37	38	39	40	41	42	43	44	45
EIGENVALUE	0.000000	0.000000	0.000000	0.000000	0.000000	0.000000	0.000000	0.000000	0.000000
DIFFERENCE	0.000000	0.000000	0.000000	0.000000	0.000000	0.000000	0.000000	0.000000	0.000000
PROPORTION	0.0000	0.0000	0.0000	0.0000	0.0000	0.0000	0.0000	0.0000	0.0000
CUMULATIVE	1.0000	1.0000	1.0000	1.0000	1.0000	1.0000	1.0000	1.0000	1.0000

	46	47	48	49	50	51	52	53
EIGENVALUE	0.000000	0.000000	0.000000	0.000000	0.000000	0.000000	-0.000000	-0.000000
DIFFERENCE	0.000000	0.000000	0.000000	0.000000	0.000000	0.000000	0.000000	
PROPORTION	0.0000	0.0000	0.0000	0.0000	0.0000	0.0000	-0.0000	-0.0000
CUMULATIVE	1.0000	1.0000	1.0000	1.0000	1.0000	1.0000	1.0000	1.0000

FINAL COMMUNALITY ESTIMATES: TOTAL = 45.501371

TM1NWF	TM2NWF	TM3NWF	TM4NWF	TM5NWF	TM6NWF	TM7NWF	TM8NWF	TM9NWF	TM11NWF	TM12NWF
0.812453	0.895754	0.821834	0.915690	0.931512	0.928759	0.774389	0.875425	0.832768	0.888151	0.774545

TM13NWF	TM14NWF	TM15NWF	TM16NWF	TM17NWF	TM18NWF	TM19NWF	TM21NWF	TM22NWF	TM23NWF	TM24NWF
0.905012	0.946672	0.958221	0.955125	0.915185	0.910118	0.790350	0.910452	0.936623	0.867982	0.918233

TM25NWF	TM27NWF	TM28NWF	TM29NWF	TM30NWF	TM31NWF	TM32NWF	TM33NWF	TM39NWF	TM40NWF	TM42NWF
0.754442	0.929327	0.878165	0.882983	0.536877	0.741542	0.936290	0.920413	0.949127	0.838870	0.909096

TM43NWF	TM45NWF	TM46NWF	TM47NWF	TM48NWF	TM49NWF	TM50NWF	TM51NWF	TM52NWF	TM53NWF	TM54NWF
0.691166	0.941540	0.897191	0.924455	0.825580	0.848926	0.909037	0.960535	0.889658	0.768556	0.838598

TM55NWF	TM56NWF	TM57NWF	TM59NWF	TM60NWF	TM61NWF	TM62NWF	TM63NWF	TM65NWF		
0.706030	0.910638	0.879444	0.795873	0.822927	0.704914	0.802710	0.758890	0.882319		

See page 3 for key.

18

Figure 9,1 All Sexual and Racial Groups Combined: Factor Weighting

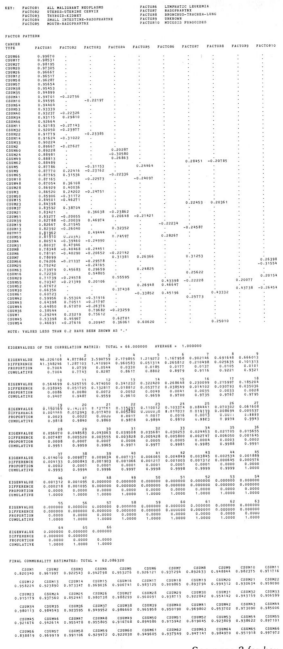

See page 3 for key.

The first four factor analyses were carried out using as variables those specific cancers which were relevant to the groups involved. In the case of white males, 50 specific cancers were used to determine the number of factors to be retained. From a scree plot of eigenvalues it could be seen that there were 10 factors which accounted for more than one unit (one percent) of variance (Figure 4,1). In total, these 10 factors could explain 78.45 percent of the variance involved. The same procedure was then used for white females to derive 10 factors which accounted for 75.81 percent of the variance. In non-white males, 10 factors were found to explain 89.03 percent of the variance, while in non-white females the comparable figure was 85.85 percent (Figures 5,1 to 9,1).

The four groups of 10 factors derived in this manner are shown in Figures 5,1 to 9,1 together with their appropriate names. From these illustrations it can be seen that the first three factors are invariably very important and will be described, therefore, in some detail. The remainder can be examined in Figures 5,1 to 9,1. In both white and non-white males, Factor I is composed chiefly of cancers of the digestive and respiratory systems and is named accordingly. This factor alone explains 25.44 percent of the variance in white males and 30.36 percent in non-white males. In white females, Factor I is mainly composed of cancers of the reproductive and digestive systems and is named for this reason. This factor accounts for 22.53 percent of the variance. In non-white females a somewhat similar Factor I explains 25.48 percent of the variance.

In all four groups, two other factors each account for at least 7.50 percent of the variance. In white males, for example, Factor II consists chiefly of skin cancers and those of the stomach and kidneys and accounts for 15.84 percent of the variance while in non-white males, Factor II is composed chiefly of cancers of the kidneys, testes and lip and accounted for 17.57 percent of the variance. In white women, Factor II incorporates mainly cancers of the bladder and urinary organs, esophagus, larynx and lungs. This factor accounts for 13.13 percent of the variance. In non-white women, Factor II includes mainly cancers of the liver and kidneys, thyroid and lungs, and accounts for 17.06 percent of the variance (Figures 5,1 to 8,1).

Factor III, in white men, mainly incorporates leukemia, other primary malignant lymphoid neoplasms, other reticuloses and cancer of the bone. It explains 7.89 percent of the variance. In non-white men, this factor is chiefly related to cancer of the bone, nose, middle ear and accessory sinuses and of the peritoneum. It accounts for 9.85 percent of the variance experienced. In white females, Factor III mainly incorporates cancers of the floor of the mouth, bronchus, trachea and lung, and the tongue. Leukemia and cancer of the bone and nervous system also contribute negatively to this factor, which in total accounted for 8.73 percent of the variance. In non-white women, Factor III consists mainly of cancer of the salivary gland, mouth, rectum and mediastinum. Cancer of the eye also contributes negatively to this factor. Together these and other incorporated variables accounted for 11.52 percent of the variance explained by this factor. In all four analyses, therefore, these first three factors were dominant, together accounting for 49.17 percent, 44.39 percent, 57.78 percent and 54.06 percent of the variance, in white men and women, and non-white men and women respectively (Figures 5,1 to 8,1).

In an effort to examine what might be termed human cancer death rates in the United States, mortality data for all four groups — white and non-white males and females — were combined. This produced a set of Pearson correlation coefficients that were essentially based on the age adjusted death rate per 400,000 in the United States. That is, they illustrated the "average" risk of cancer mortality in a group consisting of 100,000 white males and 100,000 non-white males together with equal numbers of females from both racial groups. These coefficients were then used to produce a series of factors.

The results were so unexpected that the author was advised to rerun the analysis because an error of some sort was suspected. The analysis was completely repeated, therefore, but exactly the same results were obtained (Figures 4,1 and 9,1). From these illustrations·it can be seen that in the United States, at the state level, Factor I in the human cancer analysis accounted for an enormous 60.65 percent of the variance involved in the spatial distribution. Indeed, the first three factors alone accounted for 77.50 percent of the variance experienced (Figure 9,1).

Only one logical explanation of this unanticipated result could be postulated. There must be one area of the United States where cancer mortality is very high and where the high points of numerous specific cancer distributions occur. Mortality must also decline in a fairly regular manner away from this "black spot" to reach lower levels in far distant states. Obviously, the data required mapping to test this hypothesis. It was recognized, however, that the uneven distribution of non-whites in the United States would pose a problem. For this reason, two maps were produced, one of white cancer mortality (male and female combined) and the other of total human cancer deaths (Figures 10,1 and 11,1).

As can be seen from these diagrams, the cancer "peak" in the United States is found to lie in Rhode Island, with very high total mortality in adjacent states such as Connecticut, New York, Maryland and the District of Columbia, Pennsylvania, Massachusetts and Delaware. In contrast, the lowest cancer mortality occurs in New Mexico and Idaho. Utah and Wyoming also have low mortality rates from total neoplasms, as do Georgia, Arkansas, Alabama, Mississippi, and North and South Carolina.

21

CANCER MORTALITY RATES FOR WHITE MALES AND FEMALES

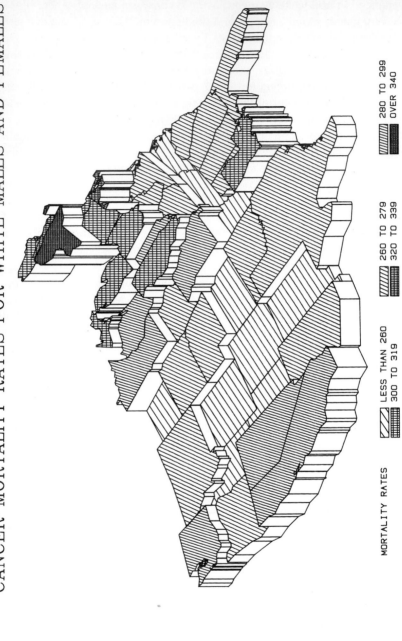

MORTALITY RATES

LESS THAN 260

300 TO 319

260 TO 279

320 TO 339

280 TO 299

OVER 340

Figure 10,1

22

TOTAL HUMAN CANCER MORTALITY RATES

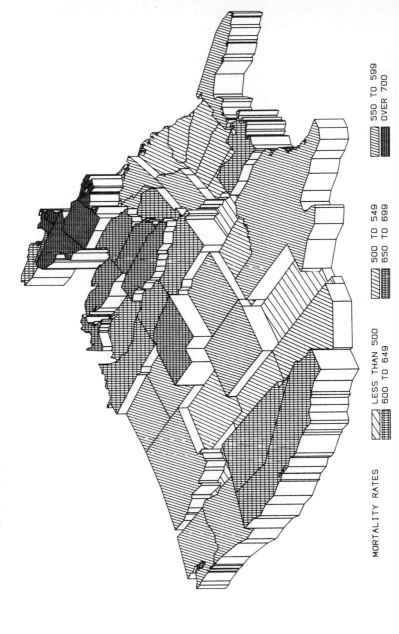

MORTALITY RATES

LESS THAN 500   500 TO 549   550 TO 599

600 TO 649   650 TO 699   OVER 700

Figure 11,1

23

Total cancer mortality, in fact, drops away to the north, west and south from the Rhode Island "peak" (Figures 10,1 and 11,1).

It follows, therefore, that there is likely to be a common cause for many specific cancers, especially those cancers that load highly on the same factor. Where the loading is negative, there may be some type of inverse relationship. Since in human cancer, three factors include most of those cancers responsible for high mortality, such as lung, breast, rectum and bladder cancer, any progress in establishing possible environmental links with them might lead to a significant reduction in the overall death rate from malignant neoplasms.[17]

CONCLUSIONS

It must be admitted that there are many possible reasons why such spatial relationships may occur. Patterns of high or low mortality may reflect exposure to varying levels of particular carcinogens for cultural, dietary, occupational or environmental reasons. Such patterns might illustrate the regionalization, for racial reasons, of a specific genetic predisposition or resistance to particular cancers. They might also graphically display geographical variations in the quality of health care, although in the United States this is not very likely. It is hardly probable that the highest death rates are associated with very poor medical services in the most densely populated parts of the country. Indeed, if anything, the reverse might be expected, for it is there that the most sophisticated treatment is often available. In addition, patterns of high or low cancer mortality could illustrate the presence, or absence, of a substance or of substances in the environment which stimulate the body's resistance to cancer. Finally, they might reflect cancer's ability to metastasize and its tendency to form secondary growths at certain preferred sites. However, it should be mentioned that even when this occurs, the selected new location might, in fact, be an organ that has been similarly damaged by carcinogens, or also lacks some protective substance. Regardless of its cause, the presence of such a total cancer "peak" is of considerable significance to the study of these associated illnesses in the United States.

REFERENCES

1. GLICK, B.J., "The Spatial Organization of Cancer Mortality". Annals, Association of American Geographers, Vol. 74(4), 1982, pp. 471-481.

2. MASON, J.T., McKAY, F.W., HOOVER, R., BLOT, W.J., and FRAUMENI, J.F. Jr., *Atlas of Cancer Mortality for U.S. Counties: 1950-1969*. DHEW Publication No. (NIH) 75-780, United States Department of Health, Education and Welfare, 1975.

3. McGLASHAN, N.D., "The Use of Cluster Analysis With Mortality Data" in McGLASHAN, N.D. and BLUNDEN, J.R., (eds.), *Geographical Aspects of Health: Essays in Honour of Andrew Learmonth*. London: Academic Press, 1983, pp. 347-360.

4. BURBANK, F., *Patterns in Cancer Mortality in the United States: 1950-1967*. National Cancer Institute Monograph 33, United States Department of Health, Education and Welfare, 1971, 594 pp.

5. *Ibid.*

6. DELURY, G.E., (ed.), *The World Almanac and Book of Facts*. New York: Newspaper Enterprise Association Inc., 1975, pp. 145-146.

7. McGLASHAN, *op. cit.*

8. McGLASHAN, N.D. and CHICK, N.K., "Assessing Spatial Variations in Mortality: Ischaemic Heart Disease in Tasmania", *Australian Geographer*, Vol. 12, 1974, pp. 190-206.

9. MASON, J.T., et al., *op. cit.*

10. BURBANK, F., *op. cit.*

11. *Ibid* and MASON, J.T., et al., *op. cit.*

12. McGLASHAN, N.D., *op. cit.*

13. MASON, J.F., et al., *op. cit.*

14. McMEIKEN, J.E., *Public Health Professionals and the Environment: A Study of Perceptions and Attitudes*. Social Science Series No. 5, Inland Waters Directorate, Water Planning and Management Branch, Ottawa, Canada, 1972, 117 pp.

15. NIE, N.H., HULL, C.H., JENKINS, J.G., STEINBRENNER, K., and BENT, D.H., *SPSS: Statistical Package for the Social Sciences* (Second Edition). New York: McGraw Hill, 1975, 675 pp.

16. JOHNSTON, R.J., *Multivariate Statistical Analysis in Geography: A Primer on the General Linear Model*. London: Longman, 1980, 280 pp.

17. BURBANK, F., *op. cit.* and PARKIN, D.M., STJERNSWARD, J. and MUIR, C.S., "Estimates of the Worldwide Frequency of Twelve Major Cancers", *Bulletin of the World Health Organization*, Vol. 62(2), 1984, pp. 163-182.

*The emerging dilemma, I believe, is not
to find and regulate a few substances,
but to deal with the hundreds and probably
thousands of substances in the human
environment for which there will be a
carcinogenic signal in some test at
some dose.*

Robert C. Barnard, 1981

The prevalance of tumorigenicity is not confined to industrial chemicals. The food chain is associated with carcinogenesis in two ways: (1) diet and (2) inherent carcinogenic components or contaminants of food.

Robert C. Barnard, 1981

2 THE SEARCH FOR CAUSAL LINKS

METHOD OF ANALYSIS:
PEARSON CORRELATION COEFFICIENT

If the cause(s) of cancer are to be discovered, links must be found between the spatial distributions of specific cancers and possible causal or protective agents. While factor analysis provides a useful method for sorting out groups of variables, other techniques of analysis are required to measure the extent and nature of the linear relationship between a dependent and one, or more, explanatory or independent variables. In the current study, Pearson correlation coefficients and stepwise multiple regression analysis were used, respectively, for this purpose. What is needed is some knowledge about how the average change in one *dependent* variable (such as a specific cancer or group of cancers) is associated with a change in another *independent* variable or variables (for example, mean annual solar radiation, or the concentration of magnesium in drinking water). Both Pearson correlation and stepwise multiple regression, therefore, provide an understanding of possible causal links between variables. The former technique, however, is limited to the examination of links between only two variables, while multiple regression is not.

DATA SOURCES

To conduct such analysis correctly, it is necessary to have medical and environmental data which relate to the same time period. Obviously it makes little sense to imply, for example, that the major increases in acid rain, which have occurred during the period 1970 and 1985, can be used to explain cancer mortality during 1950 to 1969. Nevertheless, most environmental data have been collected by water and fisheries managers, geologists, geographers, foresters, and agriculturalists for reasons completely unrelated to human health. As a result, no such synchronous environmental data sets exist. The author searched the relevant literature, therefore, and accepted for use in the following Pearson Correlation matrices and multiple regression analyses any data that had been collected before, during, or immediately after, the period covered by the mortality

29

statistics, that is 1950 to 1970. Since it is not an ideal world, this appears to be the only logical way to obtain an environmental data bank suitable for use in Pearson correlations and in multiple regression analysis. It may place some constraints on the validity of the output, but these are inevitable, if such a search for causal relationships is ever to be undertaken. One exception to this general rule was permitted. The United States Environmental Protection Agency has produced a list of hazardous waste sites which are so dangerous that they are on the Superfund priority list for immediate clean-up.[1] The chemicals at many of these sites have been dumped over a long period of time, including that covered by the mortality data. Even when this is not true, the location of these sites tends to illustrate the geographical location of the manufacture and use of toxic chemicals, in the United States. Information on the distribution of these sites was included, therefore, even though it did not fit the time criterion used for all other environmental data.

One excellent source of such environmental information is the *Water Atlas of the United States*.[2] This carries a total of 122 maps providing data on an enormous range of environmental variables. From this atlas, the author obtained data on average annual precipitation, groundwater use, hardness and sodium content of finished public water supplies and the percentage of state population drinking fluoridated water. Also used were fertilizer, DDT and phosphate application data, and information on the presence of dieldrin, lindane, cadmium, chromium, arsenic, mercury and lead in surface waters. The *Water Atlas of the United States* also included information on the use of de-icing salts by state highways departments, and the withdrawal and use of water by industry and by farmers. Figures were also given for irrigated acreage. All of this information was included in the data bank used in the Pearson correlation and multiple regression analyses. So too was data about the amount of farmland in each state, the harvested acreage of 59 principal crops; with additional detail concerning the number of bushels of barley, corn grain, oats, rye and all wheat produced. Data on cotton, hay, potato and tobacco production were also included.[3] It was felt that this agricultural information might provide clues to any relationships between the use of fertilizers, pesticides and insecticides and specific cancers. Air pollution information and other climatic data were taken from a publication by McCormick.[4]

The most comprehensive source of environmental data, however, was that published by the United States Geological Survey.[5] In 1961, the Geological Survey began a soil and regolith sampling program that was designed to give estimates of the range of element abundance in surficial materials, that were as unaltered as possible by human activity.

These were to represent the natural geochemical environment of the conterminous United States. Samples were taken at a depth of approximately 20 centimetres below the surface from locations about 80 kilometres apart, throughout the conterminous United States, and were then analyzed to determine their mineral content. In this way, 863 sample sites were chosen and the results of the geochemical analyses for 35 elements plotted on maps. The arithmetic and geometric mean, the geometric deviation and a histogram showing frequencies of occurrence of analytical values were given for each element.

On the published maps, the abundance of each element was represented by a symbol which indicated whether, at that site, the element level was very high, high, medium, low or very low, when compared with the geometric mean for the nation as a whole. These values were used by this author to generate percentage values for each state, for each level and element. For instance, in Florida 100 percent of the samples were found to be low in barium. In contrast, in Louisiana 25 percent were very low, 8.33 percent low, while 33.33 percent contained medium levels of barium and 33.33 percent had high barium levels. There were no very high barium concentrations recorded in this state.[6] Similar percentage values were calculated, for this study, for all 35 elements, for all conterminous states.

In summary, the environmental data base included details of a wide range of air and water pollutants and a variety of industrial, commercial and agricultural activities. In addition, geochemical information, which appeared to reflect, as closely as is possible, the natural chemical environment of the United States was also utilized. Details of the way in which these data were used and their original sources are found in Table 1,2.

The first step in this search for possible causal variables involved the use of Pearson correlation coefficients to explore relationships between 'natural' geochemical soil and regolith conditions and the spatial distributions of the 66 specific cancers, and cancer groups, identified at the state level, by Burbank.[7] This analysis generated 4,620 correlation coefficients. To reduce these relationships to a scale that can be easily comprehended, tables were prepared for each cancer group, for example digestive cancers, which attempted to highlight significant positive or negative correlations between particular elements and cancers (Table 2,2). Only relationships with moderate or higher correlations (r > 0.4) were included, and of these, only the most significant six appear in any of these tables, for any sexual or racial group. It should be pointed out that it is unrealistic to expect many high correlations to occur for a variety of reasons. Firstly, for most elements and their associated compounds to enter the human body they

31

must first be dissolved in drinking water, or absorbed by plants. Secondly, even if this occurs, drinking water is often boiled, causing many insoluble substances to be created. Similarly, food may alter chemically as the result of preparation, especially because of cooking. In addition, a great deal of the food consumed is grown out of state, so masking the effect of local soil conditions.

The analysis also makes the implicit assumption that population density is uniform across the United States. This is obviously erroneous. A weighting procedure was considered but rejected because the most densely settled areas usually produce virtually none of their own food, importing much of it from the surrounding rural districts. Obviously, potable water often tends to be from more local rural sources than food, since much of the latter comes from elsewhere in the United States, or from abroad. Given these difficulties, therefore, it was decided to use data from the state level that was not weighted to reflect differences in population density. For these reasons, correlations were not expected to be high. What was sought were recurring themes, or patterns, of fairly statistically significant relationships between specific cancers and elements. It was fully appreciated that in an analysis of this kind, a few high correlations might occur by chance alone, and that they would have no practical significance.

Pearson correlation coefficients were also generated to explore the relationships between the 66 specific cancers or groups of malignant neoplasms and the 65 environmental variables listed in Table 1,2. This resulted in a further 8,580 correlations. The highlights of both sets of correlations, namely those between cancer and soil elements and cancer and environmental variables are now presented.

CANCER AND THE ENVIRONMENT

Digestive Cancer

It has previously been argued that the spatial distributions of cancers of the lip, salivary gland, peritoneum and biliary passages and liver do not correlate significantly with those of the rest of the digestive system. This lack of positive association is also illustrated by attempts to explore relationships between the geochemical environment and cancer. In contrast, however, the geographical patterns of death from cancer of the tongue, floor of the mouth, and other parts of the mouth, the oral mesopharynx, the hypopharynx, the pharynx, the entire buccal cavity, the esophagus, the stomach, the large intestine, the rectum and the pancreas display major

Table 1,2 Soil and Environmental Variables Used in Pearson
Correlations and Stepwise Multiple Regression Analysis

Soil Element	How Used	Data Source
ALUMINIUM (Al)	Five Classes *(very high, high, median, low, very low)*	1
ARSENIC (As)	Five Classes	5
BARIUM (Ba)	Five Classes	1
BERYLLIUM (Be)	Three Classes *(very high, median, very low)*	1
BORON (B)	Five Classes	1
CALCIUM (Ca)	Five Classes	1
CERIUM (Ce)	Three Classes *(very high, median, very low)*	1
CHROMIUM (Cr)	Five Classes	1
COBALT (Co)	Five Classes	1
COPPER (Cu)	Five Classes	1
FLUORINE (F)	Five Classes	5
GALLIUM (Ga)	Five Classes	1
IRON (Fe)	Five Classes	1
LANTHANUM (La)	Four Classes *(very high, high, median, very low)*	1
LEAD (Pb)	Five Classes	1
LITHIUM (Li)	Five Classes	3
MAGNESIUM (Mg)	Five Classes	1
MANGANESE (Mn)	Five Classes	1
MERCURY (Hg)	Five Classes	4
MOLYBDENUM (Mo)	Two Classes *(very high, very low)*	1
NEODYMIUM (Nd)	Three Classes *(very high, median, very low)*	1
NICKEL (Ni)	Five Classes	1
NIOBIUM (Nb)	Four Classes *(very high, median, low, very low)*	1
PHOSPHORUS (P)	Five Classes	1
POTASSIUM (K)	Five Classes	1

Table 1,2 (continued)

Soil Element	How Used	Data Source
SCANDIUM (Sc)	Five Classes	1
SELENIUM (Se)	Five Classes	2
SODIUM (Na)	Five Classes	1
STRONTIUM (Sr)	Five Classes	1
TITANIUM (Ti)	Five Classes	1
VANDADIUM (V)	Five Classes	1
YTTERBIUM (Yb)	Five Classes	1
YTTRIUM (Y)	Five Classes	1
ZINC (Zn)	Five Classes	1
ZIRCONIUM (Zr)	Five Classes	1

Environmental Variable	How Used	Data Source
LAND AREA (square miles)	Unchanged	6
TOTAL AREA (square miles)	Unchanged	6
POPULATION	Unchanged	6
POPULATION DENSITY	Population Divided by Land Area	6
LOW SELENIUM IN FODDER	Unchanged (percentage of state area)	7
MEDIUM SELENIUM IN FODDER	Unchanged (percentage of state area)	7
HIGH SELENIUM IN FODDER	Unchanged (percentage of state area)	7
PRECIPITATION	Inches Per Year	8
DE-ICING SALT USE	Tonnage Divided by Land Area	8
SODIUM IN FINISHED PUBLIC WATER SUPPLIES	Four Classes	8
FERTILIZER USE	Tonnage Divided by Land Area	8
PHOSPHATE USE	Tonnage Divided by Land Area	8
DDT in 1966	Tonnage Divided by Land Area	8

Table 1,2 (continued)

Environmental Variable	How Used	Data Source
FLUORINE	Percentage of Population Drinking Fluoridated Water	8
SUNSHINE	Langleys	9
AIR POLLUTION	Suspended Particulates (Summer)	9
AIR POLLUTION	Number of Days Per Year of High Pollution Potential	9
IODINE	Prevalence Rates of Goitre in Troops - World War I	10
IODINE	Prevalence Rates of Total Thyroid Disturbance in White Selective Service Registrants - World War II	10
IODINE (LOW)	Unchanged	11
IODINE (HIGH)	Unchanged	11
SURFACE WATER HARDNESS	Parts per million	8
GROUND WATER HARDNESS	Parts per million	8
ALL HARDNESS SOURCES	Parts per million	8
POLLUTION POTENTIAL OF RIVERS	Percentage of Major State River Mileage	8
PROPORTION OF STATE FARMED	Unchanged	6
EGG PRODUCTION	Divided by Land Area	6
HARVESTED ACREAGE	Divided by Land Area	6
PERCENTAGE OF POPULATION IN MANUFACTURING	Unchanged	6
CLAY MINING AREA DISTURBED	Divided by Land Area	6
COAL MINING AREA DISTURBED	Divided by Land Area	6
STONE MINING AREA DISTURBED	Divided by Land Area	6
SAND AND GRAVEL AREA DISTURBED	Divided by Land Area	6

Table 1.2 (continued)

Environmental Variable	How Used	Data Source
GOLD AREA DISTURBED	Divided by Land Area	6
PHOSPHATE ROCK AREA DISTURBED	Divided by Land Area	6
IRON ORE AREA DISTURBED	Divided by Land Area	6
TOTAL ROCK MINING AREA DISTURBED	Divided by Land Area	6
STRIP MINING AREA REQUIRING RECLAMATION	Unchanged	6
STRIP MINING	Divided by Area of State	6
IRRIGATION WATER USE	Gallons Divided by Land Area	8
RURAL WATER USE	Gallons Divided by Land Area	8
INDUSTRIAL WATER USE	Gallons Divided by Land Area	8
IRRIGATED ACREAGE	Acreage Divided by Land Area	8
PROPORTION OF WATER FROM GROUNDWATER	Percentage of Total Use in 1970	8
BARLEY	Crop Production Divided by Land Area	6
CORN GRAIN	Crop Production Divided by Land Area	6
COTTON	Crop Production Divided by Land Area	6
HAY	Crop Production Divided by Land Area	6
OATS	Crop Production Divided by Land Area	6
POTATOES	Crop Production Divided by Land Area	6
RYE	Crop Production Divided by Land Area	6
TOBACCO	Crop Production Divided by Land Area	6
WHEAT	Crop Production Divided by Land Area	6

Table 1,2 (continued)

Environmental Variable	How Used	Data Source
CADMIUM (water)	Percentage of Tests Under 0.005 ppm	8
CADMIUM (water)	Percentage of Tests 0.005 - 0.01 ppm	8
CADMIUM (water)	Percentage of Tests Over 0.01 ppm	8
CHROMIUM (water)	Percentage of Tests Under 0.006 ppm	8
CHROMIUM (water)	Percenteage of Tests 0.006 - 0.05 ppm	8
DIELDRIN (water)	Percentage of Recorded Sites	8
LINDANE (water)	Percentage of Recorded Sites	8
ARSENIC (water)	Percentage of Sites 0.011 - 0.05 ppm	8
ARSENIC (water)	Percentage of Sites Over 0.05 ppm	8
LEAD (water)	Percentage of Sites 0.011 - 0.05 ppm	8
LEAD (water)	Percentage of Sites Over 0.05 ppm	8
MERCURY (water)	Percentage of Sites 0.001 - 0.005 ppm	8
MERCURY (water)	Percentage of Sites Over 0.005 ppm	8
TOXIC WASTE SITES	Number in State Divided by Land Area	12

SOURCES:
1. Shacklette, Hamilton, Boerngen and Bowles (1971).
2. Keller (1979).
3. Shacklette, Boerngen, Cahill and Rahill (1973).
4. Shacklette, Boerngen and Turner (1971).
5. Shacklette, Boerngen and Keith (1974).
6. Delury (1975).
7. National Research Council, Committee on Selenium (1983).
8. Geraghty, Miller, van dor Leeden and Troise (1973).
9. McCormick (1968).
10. Pendergrast, Milmore and Marcus (1961).
11. Armed Forced Institute of Pathology cited in Keller (1979).
12. Magnuson (1985).

37

		1	2	3	4	5	6
1 Lip	WM	–	–	–	–	–	–
	NWM	Ba 0.74957 0.0001 (VH)	Sr 0.56771 0.002 (H)	–	–	–	–
	WF	P 0.53602 0.0001 (VL)	Na 0.51910 0.0002 (VL)	Sr 0.51441 0.0002 (VL)	Ga 0.45988 0.001 (VL)	K 0.45253 0.0012 (VL)	Ga -0.41802 0.0031 (VH)
	NWF	Li 0.47518 0.0123 (VH)	La 0.47394 0.0125 (VL)	Y 0.40065 0.0384 (VH)	–	–	–
2 Tongue	WM	Hg 0.58782 0.0001 (VH)	Ca -0.51676 0.0002 (VH)	Sr -0.47597 0.0006 (H)	Se -0.46827 0.0008 (H)	Ni -0.42932 0.0023 (H)	–
	NWM	P -0.61325 0.0007 (H)	P -0.60308 0.0009 (L)	B 0.57995 0.0015 (VH)	Se -0.54930 0.0030 (H)	Yb 0.51955 0.0055 (VH)	Hg -0.51607 0.0059 (VL)
	WF	Li -0.44136 0.0016 (M)	–	–	–	–	–
	NWF	Mo 0.60296 0.0009 (VH)	Mo -0.60296 0.0009 (VH)	P -0.59542 0.0011 (L)	Hg -0.56367 0.0022 (L)	Ba -0.53974 0.0037 (VH)	Hg -0.53473 0.0041 (VL)
3 Salivary Gland	WM	Zn 0.43905 0.0018 (VL)	Nb -0.42574 0.0026 (VL)	Pb -0.40967 0.0038 (M)	–	–	–
	NWM	–	–	–	–	–	–
	WF	–	–	–	–	–	–
	NWF	–	–	–	–	–	–
4 Floor of Mouth	WM	Hg 0.60977 0.0001 (VH)	Hg -0.47281 0.0007 (VL)	Se -0.46709 0.0008 (H)	Al -0.45170 0.0013 (M)	Hg -0.44397 0.0016 (L)	Ca -0.42650 0.0025 (VH)
	NWM	Mn 0.62218 0.0005 (VH)	B 0.58562 0.0013 (VH)	Hg -0.56538 0.0021 (VH)	B -0.55417 0.0027 (H)	Mg -0.53017 0.0045 (VL)	K -0.52412 0.0050 (VL)
	WF	F 0.40573 0.0042 (H)	–	–	–	–	–
	NWF	Se -0.56738 0.0020 (H)	Co -0.53328 0.0042 (L)	Ga 0.47682 0.0119 (M)	Ga -0.47673 0.0119 (L)	B 0.46758 0.0139 (VH)	B -0.44397 0.0327 (VL)
5 Other Mouth	WM	Ca -0.72171 0.0001 (VH)	Sr -0.68198 0.0001 (VH)	Ba -0.55998 0.0001 (VH)	Hg -0.49455 0.0004 (H)	Hg 0.47649 0.0006 (VH)	B -0.47348 0.0007 (L)
	NWM	Be -0.60240 0.0009 (VL)	Ga 0.59235 0.0011 (M)	Zr 0.55972 0.0024 (H)	B 0.55772 0.0025 (VH)	Mn 0.51337 0.0062 (VH)	Fe 0.51766 0.0057 (M)
	WF	Na 0.78111 0.0001 (VL)	Sr 0.73500 0.0001 (VL)	K 0.72553 0.0001 (VL)	P 0.71720 0.0001 (VL)	Mg 0.65514 0.0001 (VL)	Ba 0.64796 0.0001 (VL)
	NWF	V 0.62559 0.0005 (L)	Ga 0.54313 0.0034 (L)	Pb 0.51460 0.0060 (VL)	Cu 0.50949 0.0066 (VL)	Ni 0.50578 0.0071 (L)	Co -0.48186 0.0109 (M)
6 Oral Mesopharynx (including tonsils)	WM	Se -0.55596 0.0001 (H)	Hg -0.54442 0.0001 (VL)	Hg -0.52134 0.0001 (L)	Hg 0.50743 0.0002 (VH)	Ca -0.50314 0.0003 (VH)	Sr -0.47531 0.0006 (H)
	NWM	P -0.57904 0.0016 (L)	Mg 0.55707 0.0026 (L)	Li -0.55704 0.0026 (L)	Mg -0.53856 0.0038 (VL)	Sc -0.52849 0.0046 (VL)	Mo 0.52247 0.0052 (VH)
	WF	–	–	–	–	–	–
	NWF	Na 0.72719 0.0001 (H)	Ca 0.65182 0.0002 (M)	As 0.57528 0.0017 (VH)	Se 0.55934 0.0024 (M)	K 0.55086 0.0029 (M)	Al 0.53769 0.0038 (VH)
7 Nasopharynx	WM	Na 0.50118 0.0003 (VL)	Zr -0.49987 0.0010 (L)	Sr 0.45294 0.0012 (VL)	Zr 0.44382 0.0016 (VH)	Ga 0.42313 0.0027 (VL)	Ca -0.40031 0.0048 (VL)
	NWM	P 0.73508 0.0001 (VH)	K 0.72144 0.0001 (VH)	Mg 0.63826 0.0003 (VH)	Na 0.51686 0.0058 (M)	Sr 0.50173 0.0077 (M)	Be -0.46553 0.0144 (VL)
	WF	Pb 0.42738 0.0024 (M)	Cr 0.42539 0.0026 (M)	–	–	–	–
	NWF	Be 0.66317 0.0002 (VH)	–	–	–	–	–
8 Hypopharynx	WM	Hg 0.47415 0.0007 (VH)	–	–	–	–	–
	NWM	P -0.65981 0.0002 (L)	Mn 0.63527 0.0004 (VH)	Sc 0.60722 0.0008 (H)	P 0.54114 0.0036 (VH)	Hg -0.53513 0.0040 (VL)	Fe -0.53498 0.0040 (VL)
	WF	–	–	–	–	–	–
	NWF	Mo -0.43083 0.0249 (VL)	Mo 0.43083 0.0249 (VH)				
9 Pharynx (unspecified)	WM	Hg 0.47415 0.0007 (VH)	Al -0.43265 0.0242 (VL)	Sr 0.42086 0.0029 (M)	–	–	–
	NWM	P -0.65981 0.0002 (L)	Mn 0.63527 0.0004 (VH)	Sc 0.60722 0.0008 (H)	P 0.54114 0.0036 (VH)	Hg -0.53513 0.0040 (VL)	Fe -0.53498 0.0040 (VL)
	WF	–	–	–	–	–	–
	NWF	Mo 0.43083 0.0249 (VH)	Mo -0.43083 0.0249 (VH)				- . -
10 Entire Buccal Cavity and Pharynx	WM	Ca -0.64302 0.0001 (VH)	Sr 0.60382 0.0001 (H)	Hg 0.53094 0.0001 (VH)	Hg -0.52010 0.0002 (VL)	Hg -0.50793 0.0002 (L)	Se -0.47873 0.0006 (H)
	NWM	P -0.65411 0.0002 (L)	P -0.61175 0.0007 (VL)	Mn 0.60030 0.0009 (H)	B -0.57430 0.0017 (H)	Hg -0.54583 0.0032 (VL)	B 0.54213 0.0035 (VH)
	WF	Na 0.74921 0.0001 (VL)	Sr 0.69065 0.0001 (VL)	P 0.68158 0.0001 (VL)	K 0.64316 0.0001 (VL)	Zr 0.60685 0.0001 (VH)	Ba 0.58411 0.0001 (VL)
	NWF	Ba -0.71114 0.0001 (VH)	Sr -0.61539 0.0006 (H)	B -0.54660 0.0032 (L)	Ca -0.53264 0.0042 (VH)	Hg -0.50233 0.0076 (VL)	Hg -0.48948 0.0096 (L)

Table 2,2 continues

		1	2	3	4	5	6
11 Esophagus	WM	Hg 0.59005 0.0001 (VH)	Se -0.55505 0.0001 (H)	Hg -0.52635 0.0001 (VL)	Ca -0.48143 0.0005 (VH)	Hg -0.45201 0.0013 (L)	P -0.43036 0.0023 (L)
	NWM	P -0.66431 0.0002 (L)	Se -0.60172 0.0009 (H)	B -0.55974 0.0024 (H)	Mg -0.54863 0.0031 (VL)	Hg -0.54378 0.0034 (VL)	Sr 0.53798 0.0038 (L)
	WF	Ca -0.56370 0.0001 (VH)	Sr -0.55751 0.0001 (H)	K -0.47073 0.0007 (H)	Ba -0.46146 0.0010 (H)	Ba -0.42273 0.0028 (VH)	
	NWF	Hg -0.55718 0.0025 (VL)	P -0.53064 0.0044 (L)	Ca -0.48299 0.0107 (VH)	Se -0.45663 0.0167 (H)	Hg -0.42201 0.0283 (L)	Ba -0.41980 0.0293 (VH)
12 Stomach	WM	K -0.68447 0.0001 (VL)	Na -0.67843 0.0001 (VL)	Sr -0.61357 0.0001 (VL)	Zr -0.59671 0.0001 (VH)	Ba -0.59060 0.0001 (VL)	P -0.56283 0.0001 (VL)
	NWM	Se -0.62905 0.0004 (H)	Hg -0.60889 0.0008 (VL)	Fe -0.57048 0.0019 1VL)	Na -0.55710 0.0026 (VL)	Zr -0.51158 0.0064 (VH)	K -0.50294 0.0075 (VL)
	WF	K -0.58697 0.0001 (VL)	Na -0.54415 0.0001 (VL)	Pb 0.52394 0.0001 (M)	Ba -0.51000 0.0002 (VL)	Sr -0.50811 0.0002 (VL)	K 0.50329 0.0003 (M)
	NWF	Be -0.50123 0.0077 (VL)	Fe 0.44523 0.0199 (H)	Se -0.44421 0.0203 (M)	-	-	-
13 Small Intestine (and duodenum)	WM	K 0.49061 0.0004 (M)	Pb 0.43410 0.0021 (M)	-	-	-	-
	NWM	Na 0.64284 0.0003 (L)	B 0.46332 0.0149 (VH)	Ba -0.45333 0.0176 (H)	Zr -0.44889 0.0188 (VL)	B -0.44758 0.0192 (H)	P -0.42751 0.0261 (L)
	WF	Na -0.58210 0.0001 (VL)	Sr -0.48910 0.0004 (VL)	Be -0.47806 0.0006 (VL)	P -0.45785 0.0011 (VL)	Sr 0.44538 0.0015 (M)	K -0.44196 0.0017 (VL)
	NWF	Se 0.56584 0.0021 (M)	P 0.52132 0.0053 (M)	Nb 0.48446 0.0088 (VL)	Ca 0.49089 0.0093 (M)	V 0.45124 0.0182 (L)	Pb 0.44177 0.0210 (VL)
14 Large Intestine (excluding rectum)	WM	Se -0.61023 0.0001 (H)	Be -0.57164 0.0001 (VL)	Hg 0.56623 0.0001 (VH)	Hg -0.53048 0.0001 (VL)	P -0.51223 0.0002 (L)	P -0.48700 0.0004 (VL)
	NWM	K -0.84125 0.0001 (VL)	P -0.83141 0.0001 (VL)	Mn -0.77451 0.0001 (VL)	Mg -0.72782 0.0001 (VL)	Sr -0.69828 0.0001 (VL)	Ba -0.68702 0.0001 (VL)
	WF	Se -0.66027 0.0001 (H)	Be -0.63273 0.0001 (VL)	Hg -0.56838 0.0001 (VL)	P -0.53378 0.0001 (VL)	Hg 0.53009 0.0001 (VH)	P -0.52483 0.0001 (L)
	NWF	P -0.80364 0.0001 (VL)	K -0.77131 0.0001 (VL)	Hg -0.69520 0.0001 (VL)	Zn -0.65771 0.0002 (VL)	Sr -0.65320 0.0002 (VL)	Ba -0.63640 0.0004 (VL)
15 Rectum	WM	Hg 0.61850 0.0001 (VH)	P -0.57006 0.0001 (VL)	Be -0.56919 0.0001 (VL)	P -0.56778 0.0001 (L)	Se -0.55264 0.0001 (H)	K -0.53231 0.0001 (VL)
	NWM	P -0.72369 0.0001 (VL)	Mg -0.71399 0.0001 (VL)	K -0.70469 0.0001 (VL)	Mn -0.68710 0.0001 (VL)	Ga -0.66986 0.0001 (VL)	Ba 0.61077 0.0003 (VL)
	WF	Be -0.61796 0.0001 (VL)	P -0.59152 0.0001 (VL)	Hg 0.58762 0.0001 (VH)	P -0.56489 0.0001 (VL)	Mn -0.54383 0.0001 (VL)	Zr -0.52509 0.0001 (VL)
	NWF	P -0.67126 0.0001 (L)	Mg -0.66205 0.0002 (VL)	Mn -0.65280 0.0002 (VL)	P -0.64381 0.0003 (VL)	K -0.62917 0.0004 (VL)	Ga -0.61491 0.0006 (VL)
16 Biliary Passages and Liver	WM	-	-	-	-	-	-
	NWM	Mg 0.72078 0.0001 (VH)	P 0.62861 0.0004 (VH)	Ti 0.59354 0.0011 (L)	Zn 0.56475 0.0022 (VH)	K 0.56126 0.0023 (VH)	Ca 0.55565 0.0026 (H)
	WF	K -0.65331 0.0001 (VL)	Na -0.62375 0.0001 (VL)	Ba -0.61529 0.0001 (VL)	Sr -0.54381 0.0001 (VL)	Zn -0.52532 0.0001 (P)	P -0.50560 0.0002 (VL)
	NWF	Ba 0.88308 0.0001 (VH)	Sr 0.65135 0.0002 (H)	Ca 0.50714 0.0069 (VH)	B 0.49375 0.0089 (L)	K 0.45989 0.0158 (VH)	Mg 0.41743 0.0303 (VH)
17 Pancreas	WM	-	-	-	-	-	-
	NWM	Sr -0.73485 0.0001 (VL)	P -0.72862 0.0001 (VL)	K -0.72605 0.0001 (VL)	Mg -0.72136 0.0001 (VL)	Zn -0.68138 0.0001 (VL)	Na -0.67360 0.0001 (VL)
	WF	P -0.43204 0.0022 (L)	-	-	-	-	-
	NWF	P -0.74767 0.0001 (VL)	K -0.72768 0.0001 (VL)	Sr -0.67828 0.0001 (VL)	Ca -0.66867 0.0001 (VL)	Ba -0.66727 0.0001 (VL)	Na -0.64021 0.0003 (VL)
18 Peritoneum	WM	Fe 0.40465 0.0043 (H)	-	-	-	-	-
	NWM	La -0.59888 0.0010 (H)	B -0.54679 0.0032 (M)	Zn -0.47696 0.0119 (H)	Li 0.42218 0.0247 (L)	Mg -0.40652 0.0354 (H)	Hg -0.40336 0.0369 (?)
	WF	Na 0.43748 0.0019 (L)	Sr 0.42770 0.0024 (H)	-	-	-	-
	NWF	Se 0.61086 0.0007 (M)	Ca 0.56169 0.0023 (M)	Mg 0.54265 0.0035 (L)	Fe 0.45969 0.0158 (L)	Mo 0.45447 0.0172 (VH)	Mo -0.45447 0.0172 (VL)
19 Digestive Organs (unspecified)	WM	Hg 0.47359 0.0007 (VH)	Ni 0.43696 0.0019 (H)	K 0.43409 0.0021 (L)	Sr -0.42020 0.0029 (H)	-	-
	NWM	K 0.55088 0.0029 (L)	Hg -0.51730 0.0057 (H)	Zn 0.48560 0.0102 (M)	Ba -0.46911 0.0136 (L)	Be 0.44592 0.0197 (M)	Zr 0.44139 0.0212 (H)
	WF	Sr -0.043846 0.0018 (H)	-	-	-	-	-
	NWF	As -0.51540 0.0059 (L)	Ba 0.44170 0.0211 (VH)	-	-	-	-
20 All Digestive Organs	WM	Hg 0.61576 0.0001 (VH)	K -0.55634 0.0001 (VL)	P -0.54945 0.0001 (L)	Be -0.53162 0.0001 (VL)	Na -0.52123 0.0001 (VL)	P -0.52280 0.0001 (VL)
	NWM	P -0.75117 0.0001 (VL)	K -0.74866 0.0001 (VL)	Mg -0.74162 0.0001 (VL)	P -0.70205 0.0001 (VL)	Se -0.67303 0.0001 (H)	Ga -0.67204 0.0001 (VL)
	WF	K -0.60669 0.0001 (VL)	Be -0.59493 0.0001 (VL)	P -0.59493 0.0001 (VL)	P -0.57836 0.0001 (VL)	Na -0.57305 0.0001 (VL)	Mn -0.50605 0.0002 (VL)
	NWF	P -0.84248 0.0001 (VL)	K -0.83833 0.0001 (VL)	Sr -0.73637 0.0001 (VL)	Ba -0.71273 0.0001 (VL)	Mo -0.70428 0.0001 (VL)	Na -0.68929 0.0001 (VL)

KEY: - Letters in the upper left hand corner of each cell are the generally accepted abbreviations for elements, for example, Se = selenium.
- WM = white males NWM = non-white males WF = white females NWF = non-white females
- VL = very low L = low M = medium H = high VH = very high ── concentrations of a particular element in surficial sediment or soils, as defined by Shacklette et al., 1971.

similarities which appear to reflect, at least in part, the natural geochemical environment.

It can be seen from Table 2,2 that only three of the 35 elements used in this initial analysis, namely barium, potassium and phosphorus, showed high (r $>$ 0.8, p = 0.0001) negative or positive correlations with any of the specific digestive system cancers. In addition, a further seven — beryllium, calcium, manganese, magnesium, mercury, selenium and sodium — demonstrated repeated marked (r = 0.8 to 0.6) correlation. Zinc, strontium and zirconium also displayed moderate correlations (r = 0.6 to 0.4) with some specific digestive cancer or the group as a whole.

At first glance this list appears both extensive and diverse. However, all of these substances are united by a common relationship. Potassium, phosphorus, calcium, manganese, magnesium, selenium, sodium and zinc are known bulk or trace elements.[8] Their various key roles in body functions are summarized in Table 3,2. They are present, to a varying degree, in all body fluids, tissues and bone.

In contrast, barium, beryllium, mercury and strontium are all known to be antagonistic with at least one of these bulk or trace elements, negatively influencing its ability to fulfil its necessary role. Water and acid soluble barium salts, such as carbonates, chlorides, hydroxides, nitrates, acetates, and sulphides, for example, are quite toxic. This is because the barium ion stimulates muscle tissues and causes a depression in serum potassium levels. It is generally accepted, therefore, that barium poisoning should be treated by the oral administration of magnesium sulphate solution, converting the barium to non-toxic barium sulphate. Potassium salts should also be given to elevate depressed serum potassium levels.[9] Long term exposure to excessive barium in diet seems likely to result in depressed body potassium levels.

Beryllium also has a known adverse effect on the body, accumulating in vital organs and interfering with the production of numerous enzymes. Its overriding impact is in the depletion of magnesium from the body.[10]

Mercury and selenium are known to have an antagonistic relationship. When mercury and selenium were fed together to pigs, rats and chickens, neither could later be found in the body at anticipated levels.[11] Mercury, therefore, must reduce the ability to absorb selenium in all these animals, and presumably does so in humans.

Strontium is very similar to calcium in its chemical composition and its properties are intermediate between those of calcium and barium. It is more reactive than the former, and less reactive than the latter.[12] Strontium salts, like those of calcium, are not easily absorbed by the intestinal tract.[13] When both are present, it is possible that strontium reduces the absorption

Table 3,2 Known Roles of Bulk and Trace Elements in Man

Bulk Elements	Significance
CALCIUM	Bones, teeth, blood clotting, muscle action, nerve cell communication and heart function — Key component of calmodulins — Body's most abundant mineral — Needed for parathyroid hormone function and metabolism of vitamin D — Needs magnesium, phosphorus, and vitamins A, C, D and possibly E to function correctly — Prevents too much acidity or alkalinity in blood — Muscle growth and contraction — Activates various enzymes — Needed for iron utilization and helps regulate passage of nutrients through cell walls.
IRON	Combines with protein and copper to form hemoglobin, used in oxygen transport in the blood — Necessary for myoglobin of muscle tissue — Present in enzymes that promote protein metabolism — Improves respiratory action — Synergistic with calcium and copper.
MAGNESIUM	Catalyst in utilization of carbohydrates, fats and protein — Assist in use of sodium, calcium, phosphorus and possibly potassium — Essential in bones — Counters the stimulation effect of calcium during neuromuscular contractions — Helps regulate acid-alkaline balance and utilization of vitamin B complex, vitamins C and E.
PHOSPHORUS	Synergistic with calcium in bones and teeth — Stimulates muscular contraction — Assists in utilization of carbohydrates, fats and proteins — Involved in energy production and cell repair — Essential in nucleoproteins that are responsible for cell division, reproduction and transference of hereditary traits — Kidney functioning and nerve impulse transference.
POTASSIUM	Mainly in intracellular fluids, with sodium assists in regulating water balance on either side of cell walls — Essential for normal growth, stimulates nerve impulses for muscle contraction — Preserves proper alkalinity of body fluids — Skin — Conversion of glucose to glycogen — Cell metabolism, enzymes, synthesis of muscle protein — Stimulates kidneys to excrete poisonous body wastes — With sodium helps normalize heartbeat.
SODIUM	Extracellular fluids, vascular fluids in arteries, veins and capillaries and interstitial fluids surrounding cells — Bones — Functions with potassium to equalize acid-alkaline factor in blood and regulate water balance in body on either side of cell walls — Muscle contraction and expansion and nerve stimulation — Helps increase solubility of other minerals — Acts with chlorine to improve blood and lymph health — Purge carbon dioxide from body — Necessary for hydrochloric acid production in stomach.

41

Table 3,2 (continued)

Trace Elements	Significance
CHROMIUM	Active ingredient of GTF (glucose tolerance factor) stimulates enzymes involved in metabolism of glucose and synthesis of fatty acids and cholesterol — May be involved in synthesis of protein and appears to increase effectiveness of insulin.
COBALT	Integral part of vitamin B_{12}, or cobalamin — Activates various enzymes and is necessary for red blood cells and all other body cells.
COPPER	All body tissues — Assists in formation of hemoglobin and red blood cells by facilitating iron absorption — Present in many enzymes that break down or build up tissue — Conversion of amino acid tyrosine - dark pigment of hair and skin — Protein metabolism and tissue healing — Synthesis of phospholipids, essential for protective myelin sheaths around nerves — Oxidize vitamin C, formation of elastin — Bone formation and maintenance — RNA production.
FLUORINE	Skeleton and teeth, increasing deposition of calcium, reduces tooth decay — Excess can destroy phosphotase enzyme interfering with vitamin metabolism — Antagonistic towards brain tissues — Calcium is antidote.
IODINE (IODIDE)	Functioning of thyroid gland, integral part of thyroxine, its principal hormone — Regulates energy production, promotes growth, stimulates metabolism and burning of fat — Mentality, speech and condition of hair, nails, skin and teeth effected by iodine — Assists in conversion of carotene to vitamin A, synthesis of ribosomes, absorption of carbohydrates from intestines.
MANGANESE	Activates numerous enzymes needed for utilization of biotin, thiamine and ascorbic acid — Catalyst in synthesis of fatty acids and cholesterol — Role in fat, protein and carbohydrate production — Necessary for normal skeletal growth — Possible role in blood production — Needed for formation of urea — Nourishes nerves and brain — Essential for thyroxin formation.
MOLYBDENUM	Essential part of two enzymes; xanthine oxidase used in mobilization of iron from liver reserves and aldehyde oxidase, needed for oxidization of fats — Factor in copper metabolism.

Table 3.2 (continued)

Trace Elements	Significance
SELENIUM	Protection against mercury — Body growth and fertility — Synergistic with vitamin E — Natural antioxidant appears to preserve tissue elasticity by delaying oxidation of polyunsaturated fatty acids — Necessary for prostaglandin, increases oxygen supply to heart — Antiradiation agent.
ZINC	Absorption and utilization of vitamins, especially B complex — Constituent of at least 25 enzymes involved in digestion and metabolism, including carbon anhydrase (needed for tissue respiration) — Component of insulin and needed to break down alcohol — Carbohydrate digestion and phosphorus metabolism — Synthesis of nucleic acid — Needed for growth and development of reproductive organs and prostate functioning — Healing wounds and burns — Possibly required in synthesis of DNA.

SOURCES: Kirschmann and Dunne (1984); Klayman and Copeland (1982); and National Research Council, Subcommittee on Selenium (1983).

rate of calcium, so depressing its levels in body fluids. It may also compete with calcium in various essential body functions.

The situation is rather more complex than this since many of the bulk and trace elements themselves also interact antagonistically and/or synergistically. Magnesium, for example, helps to promote the absorption and metabolism of calcium, phosphorus, sodium and potassium. Similarly, for phosphorus to be utilized effectively, there must be a specific calcium/phosphorus balance in the bones of 2.5 parts calcium to 1 part phosphorus, although phosphorus has a higher ratio in soft tissues. Potassium is commonly associated with sodium to normalize the heart beat and nourish the muscular system. Together with phosphorus, it is required to transport oxygen to the brain, while with calcium it functions in the regulation of neuromuscular activity. Zinc also plays a role in phosphorus metabolism (Table 3.2) It is clear, therefore, that the depression, or elevation, of levels of any one of these elements, either as the result of the direct impact of beryllium, barium, mercury or strontium, or because of dietary deficiencies, will have ramifications throughout the body.[14] These bulk and trace elements are so interrelated that they must obviously act together as an integrated system, the correct operation of which is likely to be essential for good health.

The complexity of the situation is further increased because the body's utilization of many of these elements is also influenced by the availability of particular vitamins. Vitamins A and C, for example, aid in the absorption of calcium; while vitamin D helps both in the reabsorption of this element in kidney tubules and in its retention and utilization.[15] In contrast, magnesium's efficiency appears to be promoted by vitamin B_6 and vitamins C and D; while manganese is most effective when ingested with high levels of vitamin B_1 (thiamine) and vitamin E.[16] Phosphorus, however, seems most available in vitamin A and D rich environments. Sodium is also most potent when taken in conjunction with vitamin D. Potassium's efficiency is promoted by vitamin B_6[17] and that of selenium by vitamin E.[18] Zinc's effectiveness, on the other hand, appears influenced by the amount of vitamins A, B_6 and E in the diet.

Alcohol is a significant antagonist of many of these vitamins and bulk and trace elements, interfering with the body's capacity to utilize vitamins A, B_1 (thiamine), B_2, B_3 (niacin), folic acid, vitamin C, D, magnesium, phosphorus and zinc.[19] In contrast, many beers and wines are extremely rich in potassium, as is coffee.[20] Smoking also lowers calcium and vitamin C levels in the body and through these, affects other bulk and trace elements. Aspirin, too, has an antagonistic relationship with several essential elements including calcium, phosphorus and potassium and with vitamins A, and B complex, B_5 (pantothenic acid) and C.[21]

Nevertheless, despite this complexity, it is apparent that the elements which correlate most highly with the spatial distribution of digestive cancers, in the United States, are united by a common thread, their ability to influence, either positively or negatively, the level of one or more of the essential bulk and/or trace elements of the body.

The significance of this fact becomes apparent after a close examination of Table 2,2. In white females and non-white males and females, liver cancer, for instance, appears to be associated with imbalances in numerous bulk and trace elements including magnesium, potassium, phosphorus, zinc and calcium. For example, high levels of calcium appear to be associated with elevated liver cancer. In contrast, in cancer of the esophagus, high calcium levels are related to low mortality from the disease. Cancer of the stomach also seems to be associated with elevated levels of many of these elements, especially potassium and sodium. It follows, therefore, that since high levels of calcium apparently inhibit esophageal cancer, yet are associated with liver cancer, mortality from these two diseases ought to have very different spatial patterns. That this is in fact the case can be seen from Figure 1,2, which allows comparison of the spatial distributing of both diseases in the United States in white females. This inverted relationship also appears to hold true elsewhere (Figures 2,4 and 4,4). It is also interesting to note that, unlike the bulk and trace elements calcium, magnesium, manganese, potassium, phosphorus and zinc, selenium always appears to play either a protective role, or be irrelevant, in the development of specific digestive cancers. Selenium seems, for example, to inhibit cancer of the tongue, mouth, oral mesopharynx, buccal activity, esophagus, stomach, large intestine and rectum, while having little or no impact on cancer of organs such as the liver and pancreas.

Possibly for this reason, the presence of mercury, in soil often appears very detrimental. Mercury, it will be recalled, has an antagonistic relationship with selenium, reducing its absorption by the body.[22] When present in the soil, in high quantities, mercury is associated with elevated mortality from cancer of the tongue, mouth, oral mesopharynx, hypopharynx, buccal cavity and pharynx, esophagus, stomach, large intestine and rectum, while being virtually irrelevant in cancer of organs such as the liver and pancreas (Table 2,2).

Since both high and low levels of the bulk and trace elements calcium, magnesium, manganese, potassium, phosphorus and zinc are associated with cancer in various specific organs, so too are barium, which depresses potassium levels, and strontium, which may reduce the quantity of calcium in serum and bones. In contrast, beryllium, which is associated with cancer of the mouth, nasopharynx, stomach and small intestine, like mercury never appears to play a positive role.

It is concluded that the evidence suggests that cancer of the digestive system seems to be related to long term imbalances of various bulk and trace elements in body fluids. These imbalances may be caused by either the direct ingestion of high or low levels of sodium, calcium, magnesium, manganese, phosphorus, potassium or zinc, or by the consumption, or absorption of high, or low, levels of substances such as barium or strontium, which interfere with the body's ability to utilize such essential elements. Selenium appears to play a unique protective role, reducing cancer mortality from many types of digestive malignant neoplasms. Since mercury is thought to reduce the body's ability to utilize selenium, it seems to have a consistently negative role, high levels of mercury being associated with various specific cancers of the digestive system

It follows that if this interpretation is correct, prediction of the distribution of high and low mortality for specific cancers of the digestive system should be possible, based on a knowledge of such factors as the mineral

45

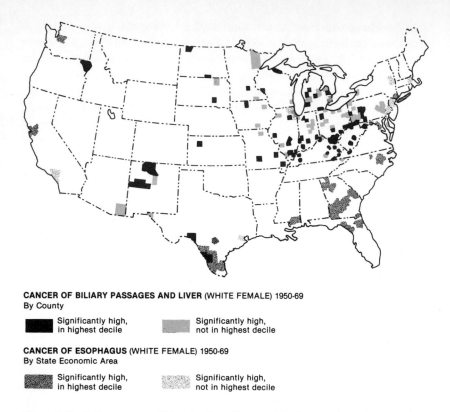

CANCER OF BILIARY PASSAGES AND LIVER (WHITE FEMALE) 1950-69
By County

■ Significantly high,
in highest decile

▦ Significantly high,
not in highest decile

CANCER OF ESOPHAGUS (WHITE FEMALE) 1950-69
By State Economic Area

▨ Significantly high,
in highest decile

░ Significantly high,
not in highest decile

Figure 1,2 A Comparison of Mortality from Cancer of the Liver and Esophagus in the United States, in White Females (1950-1969)

content of bedrock and surficial deposits, the presence or absence of bulk and trace elements in drinking water and peculiarities of diet, or levels of exposure to various substances such as barium, beryllium and strontium in the workplace. It would also follow that cancers associated with high, or low, levels of the same specific element, or groups of elements, such as calcium, are very unlikely to be present at elevated levels in the same area. For example, since cancer of the biliary passages and liver appears to be associated with very high calcium intake, while cancer of the esophagus is related to low levels of the same element in diet, it is very unlikely that both of these specific cancers will occur together at the same statistically high or low levels. In contrast, their frequencies are likely to be inversely related, unless some other overriding imbalance such as very high potassium levels stimulates liver cancer, even in calcium deficient areas.

46

While major differences in susceptibility to depressed and elevated bulk and trace elements appear to occur between the sexes and the races, overall the sum of the similarities seems to be greater than that of the differences. How many of these contrasts are the result of inherent sexual or physical characteristics, and how many result from peculiarities of diet and/or occupation is unknown. Regardless of their origin, they can be expected to cause distinct sexual and racial spatial patterns for the same specific digestive cancers. These spatial variations, however, ought to be predictable, at least in part, on the basis of known variations in susceptibility to specific bulk and trace elements. It should also be pointed out that various other elements, including aluminum, arsenic, boron, chromium, cobalt, fluorine, gallium, iron, lithium, molybdenum, scandium, vanadium and zirconium also appear to be related to the group defined as all digestive cancers by Burbank,[23] in at least one or more specific cancer(s), in a particular race or sex. The associated correlations and hence significance of these relationships was generally lower and, therefore, more likely to be due to chance than those of the elements already discussed in detail. They are listed here for the sake of completeness, in case their presence has valid medical implications.

The major environmental variables (Table 4,2) influencing mortality from digestive cancer in the United States, seem to be the use of road salt, the location of toxic waste disposal sites, population density, low selenium concentrations in crops, the distribution of sand and gravel and industrial water use. Conversely, strong sunlight is associated with low digestive cancer mortality. At first glance, this list may appear confusing, but it seems to contain three groups of interrelated variables. Firstly, high use of de-icing salts and low annual mean solar radiation are related through snowfall, which obviously influences the amount of de-icing salt put on highways and its resultant concentration in runoff. Toxic waste sites, population density, and industrial water use appear to reflect the impact of industry and, therefore, of other carcinogens in the environment. Thirdly, selenium availability tends to be low in acidic soils, such as those generally found on sands and gravels.[24]

It would appear, therefore, that the distribution of mortality from digestive cancer in the United States reflects the use of de-icing salts, low selenium levels in food and either the greater use of road salt in industrial areas, or the impact of unidentified (by this author) industrially related carcinogen(s). In white males the correlations between these variables and all digestive cancers are: de-icing salt ($r = 0.72782$, $p = 0.0001$), toxic waste site density ($r = 0.68444$, $p = 0.0001$), population density ($r = 0.66978$, $p = 0.0001$), low crop selenium ($r = 0.66268$, $p =$

0.0001), sand and gravel mining (r = 0.63764, p = 0.0001), industrial water use (r = 0.59333, p = 0.0001), and sunlight (r = −0.58313, p = 0.0001). An almost identical suite of variables seem to influence digestive cancer mortality in non-white males; industrial water use (r = 0.7584, p = 0.0001), de-icing salts (r = 0.73988, p = 0.0001), low selenium in crops (r = 0.72537, p = 0.0001), population density (r = 0.65481, p = 0.0002), toxic waste site density (r = 0.65363, p = 0.0002), and sunlight (r = −0.64859, p = 0.0003). The seven most significant environmental factors influencing digestive cancer in white females are identical to those in white males, although their ranking differs slightly. In non-white females the chief variables involved are sunlight (r = −0.73628, p = 0.0001), low selenium crop levels (r = 0.61457, p = 0.0007), de-icing salts (r = 0.58881, p = 0.0025), and industrial water use (r = 0.57193, p = 0.0018).

The relationship between digestive system cancer mortality and the use of large volumes of de-icing salt is so obvious that it requires further exploration. Each year in the United States, in the colder areas of the country, highway departments apply salts, chiefly sodium chloride and calcium chloride, to their road networks, in an effort to control the impact of snow and ice on traffic. Such de-icing salts also contain substances designed to inhibit corrosion or prevent caking. These include sodium ferrocyanide and phosphorus compounds. The use of de-icing salt on United States highways totalled more than two million tonnes during the winter of 1965-66 and its application has been steadily increasing.[25] Seventy percent of the de-icing salt used was applied in the northeast and 22 percent in the north central area. These regions contain most of the nation's highest mortality rates for cancer of the esophagus, throat, larynx, large intestine, rectum and bladder.[26]

During the winter of 1965-66, for example, Massachusetts, the District of Columbia, Pennsylvania and Illinois applied between 32 and 59 tonnes of de-icing salt per lane-kilometre. Maine, Connecticut, New Hampshire, New Jersey, New York and Vermont also used between 14 and 32 tonnes of salt per lane-kilometre on some of their highways.[27] Clearly, two million tonnes of de-icing salts dissolving in runoff from melting snow must have an impact on vegetation, soils, and the water quality in ponds, streams and wells, especially in roadside areas. Extreme fluctuations in salt concentrations are known to occur at various times of the year. In Wisconsin, for example, water at test sites was found to contain a maximum of 10,250 ppm chloride during the winter but only 16 ppm in the summer. This was not an isolated problem; during the period 1961 to 1966,

KEY TO TABLE 4,2

EN1   LAND AREA OF EACH STATE LESS WATER (SQUARE MILES)
EN2   TOTAL AREA OF EACH STATE (SQ MI)
EN3   POPULATION OF STATE (THOUSANDS)
EN4   DENSITY OF STATE
EN5   SELENIUM CONCENTRATIONS: LOW <0.10PPM, 80 PERCENT SAMPLES
EN6   SELENIUM CONCENTRATIONS: MEDIUM >0.10PPM, 50 PERCENT SAMPLES
EN7   SELENIUM CONCENTRATIONS: HIGH >0.10PPM, 80 PERCENT SAMPLES
EN8   PRECIPITATION (IN/YR)
EN9   SALT DENSITY (CONCENTRATION/LAND AREA)
EN10   SODIUM (CONCENTRATION FACTOR OF BETWEEN 1 AND 4)
EN11   FERTILIZER USE CONCENTRATION (TOTAL TONNAGE/LAND AREA)
EN12   PHOSPHATE USE CONCENTRATION (TOTAL TONNAGE/LAND AREA/)
EN13   DDT CONCENTRATION (TONNAGE/LAND AREA)
EN14   FLUORINE (PERCENTAGE WATER TREATED)
EN15   SUNSHINE (LANGLEYS)
EN16   AIR POLLUTION, SUSPENDED PARTICULATES DURING SUMMER
EN17   AIR POLLUTION, DAYS OF HIGH AIR POLLUTION POTENTIAL
EN18   IODINE, GOITRE DURING WW1
EN19   IODINE, THYROID WW2
EN20   IODINE DEFICIENCY LOW
EN21   IODINE DEFICIENCY HIGH
EN22   SURFACE HARDNESS, PPM
EN23   GROUND WATER HARDNESS, PPM
EN24   ALL HARDNESS SOURCES, PPM
EN25   POLLUTION POTENTIAL OF RIVERS
EN26   PROPORTION OF LAND IN FARMS
EN27   EGG PRODUCTION (DIVIDED BY LAND AREA)
EN28   HARVESTED ACREAGE (ACREAGE/LAND AREA)
EN29   PROPORTION OF POPULATION IN MANUFACTURING
EN30   CLAY (AREA DISTURBED BY MINING/LAND AREA OF STATE)
EN31   COAL (AREA DISTURBED BY MINING/LAND AREA OF STATE)
EN32   STONE (AREA DISTURBED BY MINING/LAND AREA OF STATE)
EN33   SAND AND GRAVEL (AREA DISTURBED BY MINING/LAND AREA OF STATE)
EN34   GOLD (AREA DISTURBED BY MINING/LAND AREA OF STATE)
EN35   PHOSPHATE ROCK (AREA DISTURBED BY MINING/LAND AREA OF STATE)
EN36   IRON ORE (AREA DISTURBED BY MINING/LAND AREA OF STATE)
EN37   TOTAL ROCKS (AREA DISTURBED BY MINING/LAND AREA OF STATE)
EN38   STRIP MINING: AREA REQUIRING RECLAMATION
EN39   STRIP MINING (RATIO OF DISTURBED TO UNDISTURBED LAND)
EN40   IRRIGATION WATER USE WITHDRAWAL (GALLONS/LAND AREA)
EN41   RURAL USE WITHDRAWAL (GALLONS/LAND AREA)
EN42   INDUSTRIAL WATER USE WITHDRAWAL (GALLONS/LAND AREA)
EN43   IRRIGATED ACREAGE (ACREAGE/LAND AREA)
EN44   PROPORTION OF GROUND WATER USE
EN45   BARLEY (CROP PRODUCTION/LAND AREA)
EN46   CORN GRAIN (CROP PRODUCTION/LAND AREA)
EN47   COTTON LINT (CROP PRODUCTION/LAND AREA)
EN48   ALL HAY (CROP PRODUCTION/LAND AREA)
EN49   OATS (CROP PRODUCTION/LAND AREA)
EN50   POTATOES (CROP PRODUCTION/LAND AREA)
EN51   RYE (CROP PRODUCTION/LAND AREA)
EN52   TOBACCO (CROP PRODUCTION/LAND AREA)
EN53   ALL WHEAT (CROP PRODUCTION/LAND AREA)
EN54   CADMIUM: PROPORTION UNDER CONC. OF 0.005 MG/L
EN54A CADMIUM: PROPORTION 0.005-0.01 MG/L
EN54B CADMIUM: PROPORTION OVER 0.01 MG/L
EN55   CHROMIUM: PROPORTION UNDER 0.006 MG/L
EN56   CHROMIUM: PROPORTION 0.006-0.05 MG/L
EN57   DIELDRIN: PROPORTION OF SITES PER STATE WHERE PRESENT
EN58   LINDANE: PROPORTION OF SITES PER STATE WHERE PRESENT
EN59   ARSENIC: PROPORTION 0.011-0.05 MG/L
EN60   ARSENIC: PROPORTION OVER 0.05 MG/L
EN61   LEAD: PROPORTION 0.011-0.05 MG/L
EN62   LEAD: PROPORTION OVER 0.05 MG/L
EN63   MERCURY: PROPORTION 0.001-0.005 MG/L
EN64   MERCURY: PROPORTION OVER 0.005 MG/L
EN65   TOXIC WASTE SITE DENSITY

Table 4,2 Pearson Correlation Coefficients: Cancers and Environmental Variables in the United States

CORRELATION COEFFICIENTS / NUMBER OF OBSERVATIONS

CORRELATION COEFFICIENTS / NUMBER OF OBSERVATIONS

Table 4,2 (continued)

CORRELATION COEFFICIENTS / NUMBER OF OBSERVATIONS

CORRELATION COEFFICIENTS / NUMBER OF OBSERVATIONS

12 states reported instances of serious water pollution caused by de-icing salts.[28]

It would appear, therefore, that states using large quantities of de-icing salts probably suffer extensive drinking water pollution from both sodium and phosphorus in wells near highways. Both of these elements have been shown to play a major role in promoting digestive cancer (Table 2,2). Why is uncertain, however one of the first technical advances in the study of chromosomes occurred when human cells were inadvertently immersed in a dilute salt solution. As a result, these cells swelled osmotically, scattering the chromosomes and allowing them to be analyzed individually for the first time.[29]

Respiratory Cancer

While the spatial distributions of cancer of the larynx, bronchus, trachea and lung (primary and secondary), and mediastinum correlate quite significantly, that of the nose shows no positive or negative relationships with the remainder of the respiratory system. For this reason, it was considered likely to have a distinct cause(s). Indeed, the distribution of cancer of the nose generally appears unique, correlating insignificantly, for example, with all other cancers in white males. While significant correlations are generally present between the spatial distributions of the remainder of cancers of the respiratory system, these tend to be weaker than those between different parts of the digestive system. In white males, for example, distribution of mortality from cancer of the larynx correlates highly with that from cancer of the buccal cavity and pharynx ($r = 0.94171$, $p = 0.0001$) and with that of the tongue ($r = 0.93671$, $p = 0.0001$), but only markedly with lung cancer ($r = 0.74369$, $p = 0.0001$) (Figure 1,1).

Under these circumstances, it is not surprising that the elements associated with cancers of the respiratory system appear virtually identical to those apparently related to digestive system cancer. This is true of all respiratory cancers, even those of the nose, except that chromium appears related to cancer of the nose in non-white females. In addition, certain metals, such as lead, appear to be linked with respiratory cancers. In general, however, cancer of the respiratory system seems to be related to the same bulk and trace element imbalances seen in digestive cancers. No high ($r > 0.8$), but 10 moderate correlations ($r = 0.8$ to 0.6) were found to exist between at least one specific cancer, or cancer of all respiratory organs, and one substance. The elements involved were barium, boron, lithium, mercury, phosphorus, potassium, selenium, sodium, strontium, and magnesium. Numerous other elements correlate with respiratory cancers at the moderate level (r = 0.6 to 0.4), calcium being particularly noticeable.

As can be seen from Table 5,2 calcium and selenium both appear to reduce mortality from respiratory cancer. Since air pollution is known to adversely influence the efficiency of vitamin E and by inference, therefore, of selenium, pollutants are likely to increase mortality from respiratory cancer, regardless of the presence of other carcinogens.[30] In addition, since cigarette smoke reduces the body's ability to utilize calcium, smoking is likely, for this reason as well as many others, to increase respiratory system cancer mortality.

High levels of barium, sodium, mercury, potassium and phosphorus all seem to be associated with elevated respiratory cancer levels. The role of these elements, therefore, would appear to be very similar in both digestive and respiratory system cancers. There is one exception, however; strontium tends to be associated with high levels of digestive cancer but depressed mortality from respiratory cancer, in certain instances, especially for non-whites. This close relationship between digestive and respiratory cancer would appear to be one of the main reasons why the major factors were able to explain such a large percentage of the variance involved in the distribution of cancer (Figures 4,1 to 9,1).

The most significant environmental variables related to high levels of respiratory cancer in the United States appear to be industrial water withdrawals, precipitation, low selenium content in fodder crops, high iodine concentrations in soils, de-icing salt use, air pollution, and toxic waste site frequency (Table 4,2). Negatively correlated variables are groundwater hardness and all sources of water hardness. There appear to be numerous links within these variables. Heavy precipitation, for example, results in elevated iodine levels. Conversely, since iodine is very insoluble in calcium and magnesium rich water, domestic supplies in hard water areas will tend to be low in both sodium and iodine and high in calcium and magnesium. Large industrial water withdrawals, the use of de-icing salts, air pollution and toxic waste site density all reflect the predominance of industry and associated carcinogens. Low selenium in local crops is also likely to be associated with a diet deficiency in this element.

White males will be used to illustrate the strength of some of these correlations: industrial water use (r = 0.57340, p = 0.0001); groundwater hardness (r = −0.56516, p = 0.0001); precipitation (r = 0.55941, p = 0.0001); all water hardness (r = −0.54908; p = 0.0001); low crop

TABLE 5,2 Cancer of the Respiratory System: Pearson Correlation Coefficients for Specific Cancers with Individual Elements

		1	2	3	4	5	6
21 Nose	WM	-	-	-	-	-	-
	NWM	Ba 0.61747 0.0006 (VH)	Sr 0.51919 0.0055 (H)	Ca 0.46548 0.0144 (VH)	Zr 0.42961 0.0253 (VL)	-	-
	WF	Zn -0.40776 0.0040 (H)	-	-	-	-	-
	NWF	Cr 0.53366 0.0042 (L)	Zr 0.51048 0.0065 (L)	Na -0.48975 0.0095 (VL)	As 0.48538 0.0103 (H)	Zr -0.47333 0.0126 (VH)	K 0.47061 0.0132 (M)
22 Larynx	WM	Ca -0.59301 0.0001 (VH)	Sr 0.57441 0.0001 (H)	Hg -0.56300 0.0001 (VL)	Ti -0.51575 0.0059 (M)	Mg 0.51292 0.0002 (VH)	Pb 0.48826 0.0098 (VH)
	NWM	B 0.68382 0.0001 (VH)	P 0.59478 0.0011 (H)	Sr 0.57925 0.0016 (L)	Hg -0.57012 0.0019 (VL)	Zr 0.56591 0.0021 (H)	Nb 0.53060 0.0044 (M)
	WF	K -0.49572 0.0003 (H)	Ca -0.49291 0.0004 (VH)	Ba -0.46920 0.0008 (H)	Ba -0.44443 0.0016 (VH)	Na 0.43943 0.0018 (VL)	Ba 0.41565 0.0033 (VL)
	NWF	Mn 0.53189 0.0043 (H)	K 0.47334 0.0126 (H)	Pb 0.45388 0.0174 (VH)	Y 0.45000 0.0185 (H)	V 0.44185 0.0210 (M)	Ba 0.41529 0.0145 (H)
23 Bronchus Trachea and Lung (primary)	WM	Na 0.45780 0.0011 (M)	Cu -0.42179 0.0028 (L)	P -0.41320 0.0035 (M)	-	-	-
	NWM	P -0.59046 0.0012 (L)	P 0.56955 0.0019 (H)	K -0.56221 0.0023 (VL)	P -0.52944 0.0045 (VL)	B 0.49156 0.0092 (VH)	Hg -0.48539 0.0103 (VL)
	WF						
	NWF	K -0.58184 0.0015 (VL)	P -0.55864 0.0025 (VL)	Sc 0.55848 0.0025 (H)	P -0.54281 0.0034 (L)	Ba -0.52801 0.0047 (VL)	Zn -0.50154 0.0077 (VL)
24 Lung (unspecified or secondary)	WM	Sr -0.53310 0.0001 (H)	Ca -0.49862 0.0003 (VH)	Hg -0.47864 0.0006 (L)	B -0.44739 0.0014 (L)	Pb -0.44412 0.0016 (VL)	Hg -0.42944 0.0023 (VH)
	NWM	Se -0.66505 0.0001 (H)	K -0.66159 0.0009 (VL)	P -0.64781 0.0003 (VL)	Hg 0.59874 0.0010 (VH)	Sr 0.59169 0.0012 (M)	Sr -0.57000 0.0019 (VL)
	WF	Sr -0.43605 0.0019 (H)	-	-	-	-	-
	NWF	P -0.68557 0.0001 (VL)	Sr -0.63102 0.0004 (VL)	K -0.61590 0.0006 (VL)	Na -0.59128 0.0012 (VL)	Zr -0.56827 0.0020 (VH)	Mg -0.55536 0.0026 (VL)
25 Mediastinum	WM	-	-	-	-	-	-
	NWM	Li -0.62383 0.0005 (M)	Co -0.58009 0.0015 (H)	Ga -0.56504 0.0021 (M)	Pb 0.52547 0.0049 (M)	Co -0.51862 0.0056 (L)	Y -0.48497 0.0104 (M)
	WF	-	-	-	-	-	-
	NWF	P 0.43226 0.0243 (VH)	Cu 0.43017 0.0251 (H)	Pb -0.41080 0.0333 (L)	-	-	-
26 All Respiratory Organs	WM	Sr -0.59208 0.0001 (H)	Ca -0.50617 0.0002 (VH)	B -0.44963 0.0013 (L)	Hg -0.42181 0.0028 (L)	F -0.42154 0.0028 (H)	Ba -0.40556 0.0042 (VH)
	NWM	P -0.70891 0.0001 (VL)	K -0.70274 0.0001 (VL)	Mg -0.61928 0.0006 (VL)	P -0.63985 0.0003 (L)	Se -0.60918 0.0008 (H)	Hg -0.60767 0.0008 (VL)
	WF	Sr -0.46447 0.0009 (H)	-	-	-	-	-
	NWF	P -0.77024 0.0001 (VL)	K -0.73593 0.0001 (VL)	Sr -0.68715 0.0001 (VL)	Na -0.66649 0.0001 (VL)	Mg -0.65346 0.0002 (VL)	Ba -0.62580 0.0005 (VL)

KEY: - Letters in the upper left hand corner of each cell are the generally accepted abbreviations for elements, for example,
Se = selenium.
- WM = white males   NWM = non-white males   WF = white females   NWF = non-white females
- VL = very low   L = low   M = medium   H = high   VH = very high —— concentrations of a particular element in
surficial sediment or soils, as defined by Shacklette et al., 1971.

54

selenium (r = 0.51965, p = 0.0002). Iodine seems most significant in white females. When correlated with goitre in First World War troops the relationship is negative (r = −0.40233, p = 0.0046). In contrast, respiratory cancers correlate positively, but at a low level, with the distribution of soil iodine (r = 0.3774, p = 0.0082).

These environmental correlations appear to confirm that high levels of iodine and sodium are associated with elevated levels of respiratory cancer, while high selenium and calcium intake seems to reduce mortality from this type of cancer. Since smoking, a known cause of lung and other respiratory cancers, depresses the body's ability to absorb calcium, there may be a significant association through this variable. Industrial air pollution also appears to play an important causal role (Table 5,2).

Cancer of the Female Genitals

The major cause of death of relatively young women in the United States is breast cancer.[31] This illness, therefore, deserves detailed examination. As can be seen from Table 6,2, in white females it appears to result from diets that are too high in phosphorus, potassium, magnesium, sodium, and zirconium. In fact, a more detailed examination of the analysis illustrates that manganese, strontium, beryllium, gallium, iron, barium, calcium and aluminum are all correlated, at least moderately (r > 0.4), with breast cancer in white females. A very similar list could also be provided for non-white women, but it would also include zinc, boron, and cobalt.

Such variety, at first glance, appears overwhelming. Perhaps it is best interpreted by accepting that breast cancer levels became elevated as the result of bulk and trace element enriched diets. This may help to explain why breast cancer is more common amongst the wealthy than the poor, and more frequent amongst women in the Developed World than those of the Developing World.[32] In the United States, breast cancer is more common in white than in non-white women; the age adjusted death rate per 100,000 being 25.29 and 22.03 respectively.[33]

Fortunately, the analysis also indicates two ways in which mortality from breast cancer might possibly be reduced. Firstly, in both white and non-white women, selenium appears to play a significantly protective role, high levels of selenium being negatively correlated with breast cancer in both cases (r = −0.52555, p = 0.0001; r = −0.63053, p = 0.0004) respectively. As might be anticipated, mercury which is always antagonistic with selenium appears to increase breast cancer mortality in both white and non-white females. Since fat is thought to elevate the body's need for selenium, a high fat diet is likely to promote breast cancer mortality,

		1	2	3	4	5	6
27 Breast	WF	P -0.60060 0.0001 (VL)	K -0.57664 0.0001 (VL)	Mg -0.57146 0.0001 (VL)	Na -0.55303 0.0001 (VL)	P -0.54643 0.0001 (L)	Zr -0.53392 0.0001 (VH)
	NWF	K -0.67005 0.0001 (VL)	Hg -0.65776 0.0002 (VL)	P -0.63455 0.0004 (VL)	Se -0.63053 0.0004 (H)	P -0.61292 0.0007 (H)	B 0.59394 0.0011 (VH)
28 Uterine Cervix	WF	Hg 0.55274 0.0001 (H)	Mg 0.47435 0.0007 (VL)	Na 0.45468 0.0012 (VL)	B -0.43633 0.0019 (L)	Ca -0.43416 0.0020 (VH)	Co -0.42401 0.0027 (M)
	NWF	Ba 0.55448 0.0027 (VH)	Ba -0.55397 0.0027 (L)	Hg 0.50617 0.0071 (L)	Sr 0.47387 0.0125 (H)	Pb 0.45865 0.0161 (L)	Hg -0.45513 0.0171 (VH)
29 Body of Uterus	WF	-	-	-	-	-	-
	NWF	Be 0.46830 0.0138 (VH)	-	-	-	-	-
30 Other Uterus	WF	Ba 0.44852 0.0014 (H)	-	-	-	-	-
	NWF	Ti 0.71850 0.0001 (VL)	Ni 0.64302 0.0003 (VL)	Nd 0.63309 0.0004 (H)	Fe 0.59816 0.0010 (VL)	Cr 0.53862 0.0038 (VL)	Co 0.53319 0.0042 (VL)
31 Uterus (unspecified)	WF	Ti -0.47798 0.0006 (VL)	Se -0.45777 0.0011 (VH)	Pb -0.46874 0.0008 (L)	B -0.44239 0.0016 (L)	Zr -0.42820 0.0024 (VL)	Nb -0.42772 0.0024 (VL)
	NWF	K -0.63147 0.0004 (VH)	Na 0.49663 0.0084 (VL)	P -0.48097 0.0111 (VH)	B 0.46181 0.0163 (VL)	Zn 0.45794 0.0163 (VL)	Mg 0.45059 0.0183 (VL)
32 Ovary	WF	Na -0.59403 0.0001 (VL)	K -0.57873 0.0001 (VL)	P -0.55274 0.0001 (VL)	Sr -0.52651 0.0001 (VL)	Mg -0.51443 0.0002 (VL)	P -0.48563 0.0005 (L)
	NWF	P -0.76648 0.0001 (VL)	K -0.75651 0.0001 (VL)	Mn -0.65505 0.0003 (VL)	Na -0.65319 0.0003 (VL)	Sr -0.64940 0.0003 (VL)	B -0.63793 0.0005 (H)
33 Other and Unspecified Genitals	WF	Se -0.51007 0.0002 (H)	Ca -0.50448 0.0003 (VH)	Hg -0.49389 0.0004 (VL)	Ca 0.44223 0.0017 (L)	Ba 0.41735 0.0032 (L)	Na 0.41681 0.0032 (L)
	NWF	Yb -0.58916 0.0012 (M)	Yb 0.52466 0.0050 (VL)	As 0.54655 0.0032 (VL)	Na -0.48929 0.0096 (H)	Ni 0.48331 0.0107 (VL)	V 0.47261 0.0128 (VL)
34 All Female Genitals	WF	Ca -0.58392 0.0001 (VH)	Sr -0.47872 0.0006 (H)	Ca 0.46756 0.0008 (L)	Se -0.44615 0.0015 (H)	Hg -0.42058 0.0029 (VL)	Zr -0.41821 0.0031 (VL)
	NWF	P -0.47590 0.0121 (VH)	Ba -0.47500 0.0123 (VL)	V -0.45722 0.0165 (VH)	Hg -0.45488 0.0171 (VH)	Sr -0.43305 0.0240 (M)	-

KEY: - Letters in the upper left hand corner of each cell are the generally accepted abbreviations for elements, for example,
Se = selenium.
- WF = white females   NWF = non-white females
- VL = very low   L = low   M = medium   H = high   VH = very high —— concentrations of a particular element in
surficial sediment or soils, as defined by Shacklette et al., 1971.

especially in selenium deficient areas. Amongst the 65 environmental variables, the strongest breast cancer correlations are with the amount of de-icing salt used on highways (r = 0.66412, p = 0.0001) and the distribution of forage and grain crops that are low in selenium (r = 0.61517, p = 0.0001) (Table 4,2).

There is also a moderate negative correlation between breast cancer and sunlight. High exposure to sunlight, therefore, might play a role in preventing breast cancer (r = −0.59869, p = 0.0001). Because of this apparent relationship, regions of significantly high breast cancer and melanoma mortality appear reversed and are separated, in the United States, by the isopleth which represents 375 langleys of mean daily radiation (Figure 3,1). Why this relationship may occur is unclear, but sunlight is involved in the production of vitamin D by the body, which aids in the absorption of calcium.

Vitamin D also modifies the effectiveness of vitamin A.[34] Naturally, because of these and other synergistic and antagonistic relationships, vitamin D tends to influence virtually all other trace elements and vitamin levels in the body.

In stark contrast to breast cancer, that of the uterine cervix appears to be related in white women to bulk element deficiencies, namely of magnesium, sodium and calcium (Table 6,2). In non-white women, barium, which depresses potassium levels in the body, and strontium, which probably reduces the effectiveness of calcium, appear to be associated with elevated mortality from cancer of the uterine cervix. Selenium seems to have no impact on mortality from this disease (Table 6,2).

Cancer of the body of the uterus has a very different spatial distribution from either breast cancer or cancer of the uterine cervix. In white females there is no reliable coefficient of correlation ($r > 0.4$), either positive or negative, with any soil element. There is only one exception to this rule. In non-white women very high levels of beryllium correlates moderately with cancer of the body of the uterus ($r = 0.46830$, $p = 0.0138$). However, amongst the environmental variables the situation is reversed, with the amount of land devoted to hay growth correlating, either markedly or highly, with the incidence of cancer of the body of the uterus (Table 4,2). In white females, for example, the relationship is marked ($r = 0.68591$, $p = 0.0001$), while in non-white women the correlation is high, indeed one of the highest found in this attempt to discover possible causal cancer variables ($r = 0.84755$, $p = 0.0001$). In non-white women there is also a marked positive correlation with oat acreage ($r = 0.79001$, $p = 0.0001$). The only reasonable conclusion to draw from this analysis would appear to be that cancer of the body of the uterus is not associated with the elevation or depression of dietary bulk or trace elements, like most other cancers, but rather it is more likely to be related to (a) specific carcinogen(s) that are used in farming, particularly in the cultivation of hay and oats. Unfortunately, the author only has detailed information on the use of a limited number of fertilizers, pesticides and insecticides in the United States. From this restricted data base, it appears that cancer of the body of the uterus is not significantly related to the use of DDT, lindane, dieldrin, nitrates or phosphates.

There also appears to be very little correlation in white women between bulk and trace elements in the soil and other uterine cancers, such as choriomepithelioma and chorionic carcinoma. In non-white women, however, these cancers seem to be associated with low exposure to several metals including titanium, nickel, iron, chromium and cobalt. Farming appears to play no role in the origin of these illnesses.

In contrast, cancer of the ovary, like that of the breast, seems to be related to a number of bulk and trace element excesses, such as too much sodium, phosphorus, potassium and manganese. In addition, strontium may play a negative role (Table 6,2). The analysis of relationships between cancer of all female genitals and soil bulk and trace elements tends to suggest that calcium and selenium both play a protective role, while strontium, barium, mercury and zirconium are possibly carcinogens.

Cancer of the Male Genitals

High levels of strontium seem to be associated with genital cancers in non-white males, while high levels of calcium appear to be protective against prostate cancer, but not against cancer of the testes, where they may even promote it. Barium also appears to be a protective agent for non-white males against cancer of the prostate and testes, and, as a result, against all cancer of the male genital organs. Unfortunately barium, the potassium depressant, does not seem to play the same beneficial role in white males. High calcium levels also appear to be associated with genital cancer in white males (Table 7,2).

Cancer of the Kidney, Bladder and Urinary Tract

Cancer of the kidney appears to be associated with elevated levels of several bulk and trace elements and their antagonists, namely sodium, calcium, magnesium, potassium, phosphorus, strontium and barium (Table 8,2). Zinc, gallium and manganese appear to be of lesser significance. While the exact nature of these relationships varies with both race and sex, such elements seem to play common roles. Under these circumstances, one might expect cancer of the kidney to be spatially associated with other cancers that are possibly associated with an imbalance of similar bulk and trace elements. It should also be noted that high levels of zirconium, for some unknown reason, appear to be linked to reduced mortality from this disease, while selenium seems to play only a very minor protective role.

Very different soil elements correlate with the spatial distribution of cancer of the bladder and urinary organs. Selenium and mercury, for example, are far more related to the disease, selenium apparently being a protective element and mercury the reverse. Also of note is the apparently

TABLE 7,2   Cancer of the Male Genitals: Pearson Correlation Coefficients for Specific Cancers with Individual Elements

		1	2	3	4	5	6
27 Breast	WM	Zr -0.43192 0.0022 (VH)	Mg -0.42463 0.0026 (VL)	-	-	-	-
	NWM	Ti -0.68305 0.0001 (M)	Yb -0.59215 0.0011 (M)	Nd -0.55005 0.0030 (VL)	Nb -0.53914 0.0037 (L)	Yb 0.52293 0.0051 (VH)	La 0.49765 0.0083 (VH)
35 Prostate	WM	Zr 0.46448 0.0009 (L)	Ca -0.42385 0.0027 (VL)	B -0.41358 0.0320 (L)	-	-	-
	NWM	Ba -0.84012 0.0001 (VH)	Sr -0.64292 0.0003 (H)	Na -0.58276 0.0014 (VH)	Ca -0.56378 0.0022 (VH)	Sr -0.53096 0.0044 (VH)	Hg -0.48073 0.0111 (L)
36 Testis	WM	P -0.49316 0.0004 (VL)	Mg -0.49222 0.0004 (VL)	Sr -0.48193 0.0005 (VL)	Ba 0.46801 0.0008 (VL)	Mn 0.46457 0.0009 (VH)	Zn 0.46321 0.0009 (H)
	NWM	Ba 0.88418 0.0001 (VH)	Sr 0.66666 0.0001 (H)	Ga 0.54333 0.0034 (H)	Ca 0.50588 0.0071 (VH)	B 0.47187 0.0130 (L)	Na 0.44108 0.0213 (H)
37 Other Male Genitals	WM	-	-	-	-	-	-
	NWM	Mn 0.64408 0.0003 (VL)	Na 0.63583 0.0004 (VL)	Ba 0.62763 0.0005 (VL)	Nd 0.60979 0.0007 IVH)	Zr 0.56640 0.0021 (VH)	Sr 0.55709 0.0026 (VL)
38 All Male Genital Organs	WM	Zr 0.46790 0.0008 (L)	Ca -0.44031 0.0017 (VL)	-	-	-	-
	NWM	Ba -0.80968 0.0001 (VH)	Sr 0.63463 0.0004 (H)	Na -0.60718 0.0008 (VH)	Ca -0.56792 0.0020 (VH)	Sr 0.54485 0.0033 (VH)	Nb -0.49415 0.0088 (L)

KEY: – Letters in the upper left hand corner of each cell are the generally accepted abbreviations for elements, for example,
       Se = selenium.
     – WM = white males   NWM = non-white males
     – VL = very low   L = low   M = medium   H = high   VH = very high —— concentrations of a particular element in
       surficial sediment or soils, as defined by Shacklette et al., 1971.

protective roles played by calcium, barium and strontium. In white females, for example, there is a moderate negative correlation between mortality from bladder and urinary cancer and very high soil calcium content (r = −0.51573, p = 0.0002). Cancer of the bladder, therefore, appears to have more in common with cancers of the digestive system (Table 2,2) than with that of the kidney (Table 8,2).

Environmental variables that appear related to the distribution of cancer of the kidney, in white males, include road salt use and exposure to possible agricultural carcinogens (Table 4,2). In addition, cancer of the kidney appears inversely related to exposure to sunlight (r = −0.50649, p = 0.0002). In non-white males and females, depressed iodine soil levels also appear to be important. In white females, exposure to agricultural carcinogens seem significant, while sunlight is again perhaps protective (r = −0.48658, p = 0.0005). In white males and females and non-white males, high mortality from cancer of the bladder and other urinary organs appears most related to low selenium levels in fodder crops and to the use of de-icing salts on highways. In non-white females, coal mining and air pollution are apparently of particular significance, although the disease also appears to be promoted by low selenium content in fodder (Table 4,2).

59

TABLE 8.2   Cancer of the Kidney, Bladder and Urinary Organs: Pearson Correlation Coefficients for Specific Cancers with Individual Elements

		1	2	3	4	5	6
39 Kidney	WM	Na -0.65930 0.0001 (VL)	Zr -0.58908 0.0001 (VH)	Sr -0.58615 0.0001 (VL)	P -0.58292 0.0001 (VL)	K -0.58159 0.0001 (VL)	Mg -0.56126 0.0001 (VL)
	NWM	Ba 0.66767 0.0001 (VH)	Na -0.62622 0.0005 (VL)	Sr -0.61429 0.0007 (VL)	K -0.59875 0.0010 (VL)	Zr -0.59559 0.0011 (VH)	P -0.58968 0.0012 (VL)
	WF	Na 0.54176 0.0001 (M)	Sr 0.51947 0.0002 (H)	Sr -0.47446 0.0007 (VL)	K -0.46782 0.0008 (VL)	Na -0.46623 0.0008 (VL)	Ca -0.45678 0.0011 (VL)
	NWF	Mg 0.68914 0.0001 (VH)	Sr -0.65788 0.0002 (VL)	P -0.65032 0.0002 (VL)	K -0.64627 0.0003 (VL)	Na -0.62983 0.0004 (VL)	Mg -0.61765 0.0006 (VL)
40 Bladder and Other Urinary Organs	WM	Be -0.56785 0.0001 (VL)	Zr -0.51145 0.0002 (VH)	Hg 0.53598 0.0001 (VH)	Ni -0.49699 0.0003 (H)	P -0.48904 0.0004 (VL)	P -0.47516 0.0006 (L)
	NWM	P -0.56211 0.0023 (L)	Hg 0.51628 0.0058 (VH)	Hg -0.51458 0.0060 (VL)	K -0.50275 0.0075 (VL)	Zr -0.50046 0.0079 (VH)	Se -0.49057 0.0094 (H)
	WF	Ca -0.51573 0.0002 (VH)	Be -0.48755 0.0004 (VL)	Sr -0.46325 0.0009 (H)	Hg -0.42003 0.0030 (VL)	F -0.41449 0.0034 (H)	Be 0.40055 0.0048 (VH)
	NWF	Ba -0.53037 0.0044 (VH)	Hg -0.50840 0.0068 (L)	Hg -0.47587 0.0121 (VL)	Sr 0.49164 0.0092 (L)	Mo 0.47113 0.0131 (VH)	Mo -0.47113 0.0131 (VL)
41 All Urinary Tract Organs	WM	Be -0.56532 0.0001 (VL)	Zr -0.56531 0.0001 (VH)	P -0.54620 0.0001 (VL)	Hg 0.53895 0.0001 (VH)	Na -0.51534 0.0002 (VL)	P -0.50838 0.0002 (L)
	NWM	K -0.67495 0.0001 (VL)	Zr -0.67163 0.0001 (VH)	P -0.65074 0.0002 (VL)	Na -0.64382 0.0003 (VL)	Sr -0.64341 0.0003 (VL)	Mg -0.59808 0.0010 (VL)
	WF	Be -0.53718 0.0001 (VL)	Se -0.51753 0.0002 (H)	P -0.50080 0.0003 (L)	Hg -0.43173 0.0022 (VL)	Zr -0.40582 0.0042 (VH)	-
	NWF	K -0.71149 0.0001 (VL)	P -0.68008 0.0001 (VL)	Mn -0.65385 0.0002 (VL)	Zr -0.65206 0.0002 (VH)	Ba -0.58810 0.0013 (VL)	Mg -0.56808 0.0020 (VL)

KEY: - Letters in the upper left hand corner of each cell are the generally accepted abbreviations for elements, for example, Se = selenium.
- WM = white males   NWM = non-white males   WF = white females   NWF = non-white females
- VL = very low   L = low   M = medium   H = high   VH = very high —— concentrations of a particular element in surficial sediment or soils, as defined by Shacklette et al., 1971.

Cancer of the Integument

It is widely believed by epidemiologists, and indeed the general public, that there is a clear causal relationship between overexposure to sunlight and the incidence of malignant melanoma of the skin.[35] However, when the global distribution of this illness is reviewed this supposed relationship is found to be associated with numerous anomalies and internal inconsistencies. Melanoma is infrequent in pigmented races, including those of Asia, and its incidence does not vary with latitude amongst them. The disease shows a relative predilection for the feet of pigmented races, a strange site for a cancer supposedly caused by overexposure to the sun. Similarly, within the United Kingdom, Scotland has higher mortality rates from melanoma than either England or Wales. In the rest of Europe, there are comparatively high rates in Switzerland, Hungary, Romania, France and the north of Italy (latitudes 45° to 48° north). Rates of the incidence of melanoma then tend to fall, between latitudes 48° and 55° north, yet they rise again in Finland, Denmark, Norway and Sweden, a distribution pattern very inconsistent with simple overexposure to sunlight as an overriding cause.[36]

It has also been established that in North America, neither latitude nor altitude appear to correlate highly with melanoma mortality. Even when attempts are made to express the effects of latitude in terms of received ultraviolet radiation, the resulting index does not correlate very strongly with melanoma mortality (r = 0.67 in males and 0.56 in females).[37]

The geographical gradients of melanoma in Australia are also contradictory. Within Queensland, which spans 19 degrees of latitude, there seems to be higher incidence rates on the coast than inland.[38] Yet there is little difference, in age-standardized melanoma incidence, between northern and southern coastal regions, despite major variations in daily average hours of sunshine.[39] In Western Australia, a state spanning 21 degrees of latitude, melanoma appears appreciably lower in the north, that is nearer to the equator, than in the south.[40]

When socio-economic factors are examined, it is found that melanoma is more common amongst the rich than the poor.[41] Yet this group is perhaps least likely to work outdoors in activities such as agriculture. Indeed, melanoma is paradoxically most common in those who work indoors.[42] Similarly, dietary habits appear to be related to the incidence of melanoma, with Hawaiian whites, Jews living in Israel and the Spanish populations of New Mexico, Navarra and Zaragoza having particularly low rates, for the latitudes involved.

The author is sorry to belabor the point that melanoma is very unlikely to be related simply to overexposure to sunlight, but when something that is so obviously erroneous is so widely believed, it tends to obscure the truth. In the United States, for example, Arizona and New Mexico receive the most solar radiation, yet melanoma mortality for males, in large areas of these states, is significantly lower than the national average.[43] In the present analysis, it was found that, in white males, nine environmental variables correlated either positively or negatively with melanoma mortality rates more highly than exposure to sunlight. Fifteen variables did the same in the case of white females. For non-whites, both male and female, exposure to sunlight was totally irrelevant. Similarly, since the correlation between sunlight and melanoma in white males (r = 0.4339, p = 0.0021) and white females (r = 0.31638, p = 0.0285) was relatively low, the distributions of numerous soil elements also correlated more highly with this specific cancer than did exposure to the sun (Table 9,2).

In white males, melanoma mortality in the United States, appears more related to excesses of iodine in diet than to overexposure to sunlight. In areas of high iodine content, for instance, the relationship is positive (r = 0.54292, p = 0.0001). In areas of low iodine content the association

TABLE 9,2 Cancer of the Entire Integument: Pearson Correlation Coefficients for Specific Cancers with Individual Elements

		1	2	3	4	5	6
42 Melanoma	WM	K 0.65729 0.0001 (VL)	Na 0.64416 0.0001 (VL)	P 0.59918 0.0001 (VL)	Ba 0.57827 0.0001 (L)	Sr 0.57206 0.0001 (VL)	Na -0.50234 0.0003 (M)
	NWM	La -0.57288 0.0018 (H)	Yb 0.46358 0.0149 (M)	Hg -0.46334 0.0149 (L)	As 0.44066 0.0214 (H)	Sr 0.42974 0.0252 (M)	Zr 0.41699 0.0305 (L)
	WF	Na 0.71150 0.0001 (VL)	K 0.71075 0.0001 (VL)	P 0.68406 0.0001 (VL)	Sr 0.66744 0.0001 (VL)	Zr 0.66486 0.0001 (VH)	Mg 0.58402 0.0001 (VL)
	NWF	Yb -0.56055 0.0024 (L)	Ba -0.50899 0.0067 (VH)	B -0.50089 0.0078 (L)	-	-	-
43 Skin	WM	Na 0.67001 0.0001 (VL)	Zr 0.62653 0.0001 (VH)	P 0.61916 0.0001 (VL)	Sr 0.60103 0.0001 (VL)	Ga 0.59480 0.0001 (VL)	Mg 0.59433 0.0001 (VL)
	NWM	As -0.60921 0.0008 (H)	Ca -0.58492 0.0014 (M)	K -0.57127 0.0019 (VL)	Li -0.57046 0.0019 (H)	Na -0.52752 0.0047 (M)	Co 0.51439 0.0061 (H)
	WF	Na 0.76332 0.0001 (VL)	Sr 0.71255 0.0001 (VL)	P 0.70371 0.0001 (VL)	Zr 0.68746 0.0001 (VH)	Mg 0.68473 0.0001 (VL)	K 0.67333 0.0001 (VL)
	NWF	Ba 0.60237 0.0009 (VH)	Ca -0.55657 0.0026 (VH)	Sr -0.54083 0.0036 (H)	Co -0.48929 0.0096 (M)	Zr 0.45141 0.0181 (VH)	Sr -0.43175 0.0245 (VH)
44 Entire Integument	WM	Na 0.69411 0.0001 (VL)	K 0.64523 0.0001 (VL)	P 0.64296 0.0001 (VL)	Sr 0.62028 0.0001 (VL)	Zr 0.60766 0.0001 (VH)	Ga 0.58331 0.0001 (VL)
	NWM	La -0.55101 0.0029 (H)	Co -0.52028 0.0054 (H)	Nb -0.48425 0.0105 (VL)	La 0.45709 0.0165 (VH)	Ca -0.45098 0.0182 (M)	Ca 0.44862 0.0189 (VL)
	WF	Na 0.79223 0.0001 (VL)	P 0.74406 0.0001 (VL)	Sr 0.74108 0.0001 (VL)	K 0.73936 0.0001 (VL)	Zr 0.72520 0.0001 (VH)	Mg 0.68411 0.0001 (VL)
	NWF	Ba -0.65211 0.0002 (VH)	Sr -0.52223 0.0052 (H)	Ca -0.48666 0.0100 (VH)	Na -0.48341 0.0106 (M)	Sr -0.41593 0.0309 (VH)	K -0.40619 0.0355 (VH)

KEY: – Letters in the upper left hand corner of each cell are the generally accepted abbreviations for elements, for example, Se = selenium.
– WM = white males   NWM – non-white males   WF = white females   NWF = non-white females
– VL = very low   L = low   M = medium   H = high   VH = very high── concentrations of a particular element in surficial sediment or soils, as defined by Shacklette et al., 1971.

is reversed (r = −0.54292, p = 0.0001). High water hardness is also associated with low melanoma mortality. However, since iodine declines in solubility with hardness, this relationship (r = −0.51696, p = 0.0002) is explicable. Very similar correlations also occur in the case of white women, although the levels are somewhat lower. Mortality from melanoma for whites, in the United States, also appears to be related to deficiencies of certain other elements. These include barium, gallium, potassium, magnesium, manganese, sodium, phosphorus, strontium, and zinc. Melanoma, therefore, appears to be a cancer that is strongly associated with low levels of a variety of bulk and trace elements and their antagonists, in diet (Table 9,2).

Nevertheless, there is clearly some relationship between melanoma and exposure to sunlight (Table 4,2). It is suggested, therefore, that high levels of iodine and low levels of most of the major bulk and trace elements may increase the susceptibility of white skin to damage from ultraviolet radiation. Why this may occur is unknown to this author. If this hypothesis is correct then, melanoma, in white women, occurs for reasons that are virtually the reverse of those that seem associated with breast cancer development.

TABLE 10,2   Cancer of the Eye and Nervous System: Pearson Correlation Coefficients for Specific Cancers with Individual Elements

		1	2	3	4	5	6
45 Eye	WM	Be 0.44714 0.0014 (VL)	Mg 0.41052 0.0038 (VL)	-	-	-	-
	NWM	Se 0.58285 0.0014 (H)	Na -0.48004 0.0113 (H)	P 0.46079 0.0156 (L)	V -0.45605 0.0168 (M)	Mg 0.45031 0.0184 (VL)	Ga -0.44697 0.0194 (H)
	WF	Hg 0.45327 0.0012 (L)	Hg 0.41832 0.0031 (VL)	-	-	-	-
	NWF	Yb 0.48528 0.0103 (L)	Cu 0.44831 0.0190 (VL)	As 0.44670 0.0195 (VL)	Nb 0.41890 0.0296 (VL)	Al 0.40406 0.0366 (M)	-
46 Nervous System	WM	Ba -0.42251 0.0028 (VH)	-	-	-	-	-
	NWM	Ba 0.63799 0.0003 (VH)	Na -0.58857 0.0013 (VL)	K -0.56814 0.0020 (VL)	P -0.56139 0.0023 (VL)	K 0.53495 0.0041 (H)	Sr -0.52353 0.0051 (VL)
	WF	As 0.46494 0.0009 (VL)	Yb 0.40304 0.0045 (VL)	-	-	-	-
	NWF	Fe 0.60009 0.0009 (L)	Ba -0.59199 0.0012 (VH)	Ca 0.49760 0.0083 (M)	Na -0.47037 0.0133 (VL)	P -0.48487 0.0104 (L)	Zn -0.46929 0.0135 (VL)

KEY: - Letters in the upper left hand corner of each cell are the generally accepted abbreviations for elements, for example,
   Se = selenium.
   - WM = white males   NWM = non-white males   WF = white females   NWF = non-white females
   - VL = very low   L = low   M = medium   H = high   VH = very high —— concentrations of a particular element in
   surficial sediment or soils, as defined by Shacklette et al., 1971.

One would expect, therefore, an inversion of mortality rates from these two diseases. This seems to be true of the United States (Figure 3,1).

Skin cancer is the term used by Burbank[44] to describe all other cancers of the skin, excluding melanoma and genital organ cancer. In white males in the United States there is a band of decreased death rates from skin cancer across the northern third of the country, and a cluster of increased mortality rates in the south and south midwest. Increased mortality rates are also found in the south and south midwest for white females, while lower death rates occur in the northeast, north midwest and along the west coast.

Skin cancer, like melanoma, appears to be connected with high iodine intake. However, the relative significance of other bulk and trace elements differs markedly; so that the spatial distributions of the two illnesses should not be expected to be particularly similar. In skin cancer, the key associated elements are sodium, strontium, potassium, magnesium and calcium. While deficiencies of these elements also appear to be linked with melanoma, low levels of calcium seems more significant in skin cancer. There are similarities, however, since in whites, high zirconium levels in soils correlate significantly with elevated levels of both illnesses. Perhaps the biggest difference, though, is that skin cancer, unlike melanoma, shows no evidence of any connection with sunlight. In white males and white females the correlation is low (r = 0.39248, p = 0.0058 and r = 0.20193, p = 0.1687 respectively). The United States distribution patterns appear to be related to high levels of road salt use, which for this particular cancer are protective, and elevated iodine and bulk and

63

trace element deficiencies, found in the soils of the unglaciated south and southwest. Selenium appears to give very little protection against either melanoma or skin cancer. Mercury, therefore, is also unrelated to their distribution.

Mortality from cancer of the entire integument occurs in three bands, with decreased rates in the north, average central and elevated death rates in the south of the United States. These divisions apparently reflect the glacial history of North America. Newer, glacially derived soils, in the northern areas are iodine poor, but relatively rich in sodium, potassium, phosphorus and strontium. Soils in the south, in contrast, are generally much older, more deeply weathered and depleted of many bulk and trace elements. Iodine levels are high, however.[45] So, too, is sunlight, which apparently plays a role in melanoma, but only when certain mineral deficiencies are present in diet.

Cancer of the Eye and Nervous System

Cancer of the eye and optic nerve, together with all malignant neoplasms of the brain, spinal cord, cauda equina and all other nerves are included in this category.[46] Cancer of the eye is a rare disease in the United States. It is, however, more common in white males than in any other group. For such individuals there is a small cluster of increased death rates in Tennessee and North Carolina.[47] Cancer of the nervous system, in white males, is also commonest in the south and in California.[48]

It can be seen from Table 10,2 that the group of bulk and trace elements that normally appear to be closely associated with most cancers play only a small role in cancer of the eye. Indeed, high soil selenium, which is almost universally protective, correlates positively with cancer of the eye in non-white males ($r = 0.58285$, $p = 0.0014$). In contrast, several environmental variables show some links to cancer of the eye. In particular it was seen to be related to cotton and tobacco cultivation in white males ($r = 0.56244$, $p = 0.0151$; $r = 0.53447$, $p = 0.0271$) (Table 4,2).

Cancer of the remainder of the nervous system was found to be linked to a variety of apparently unrelated elements. This is possibly because the category includes so many distinct cancer sites. Only in non-white males was there a very clear picture. In this group, cancer of the nervous system appears to be associated with too much sodium, potassium, phosphorus and strontium. In addition, there was a high correlation between this type of malignant neoplasm and iodine, all four indicators of this element placing in the highest positions in the ranked Pearson correlation coefficient tables (Table 4,2). The distribution of goitre amongst World

War I troops, for example, displayed a high correlation (r = 0.82207, p = 0.0001) with cancer of the nervous system, in non-white males, which is, therefore, thought to be related to an iodine deficiency. In white males, the highest correlation found was with cotton cultivation (r = 0.49382, p = 0.0373). In non-white females the strongest correlation was with road salt use (r = 0.64864, p = 0.0006).

In summary, there is some suggestion that cancer of the eye and nervous system, in white males, may be due to exposure to agricultural carcinogen(s), however the evidence is weak. In non-white males, cancer of the nervous system appears to be associated with an iodine deficiency and with too much sodium, potassium, phosphorus and strontium. These elements may also play a similar role in non-white women.

Cancer of the Thyroid and Bone Cancer

In both white women and men, the three major elements associated with thyroid cancer appear to be barium, sodium and potassium (Table 11,2). Since both barium and sodium are potassium antagonists, and cause depressed potassium levels in body serum, it would appear likely that thyroid cancer is related in some way to a potassium imbalance.

If this hypothesis is correct, the well-known association between goitre and thyroid cancer becomes understandable.[49] Since the incidence of both goitre and thyroid cancer tend to peak in the same regions, it was initially believed that they had a common cause. However, it was then discovered that goitre could be treated successfully with iodine.[50] To reduce the incidence of this disease, potassium iodide was added to table salt.' As a consequence, the incidence of goitre dropped markedly in the United States. Yet surprisingly, mortality from thyroid cancer actually increased steadily over the same period, that is from 1939 to 1955.[51]

It would appear that the addition of iodized salt to food resulted in the absorption of more sodium, potassium and iodine. The iodine apparently prevented goitre, while the sodium and potassium, as expected from Table 11,2, became associated with elevated levels of thyroid cancer. Strangely enough, the situation is different in non-whites where there is a very clear correlation between thyroid cancer and iodine deficiency. In non-white males there are marked correlations (both negative and positive) between the four environmental variables that indicated the presence of iodine, in the environment, and thyroid cancer. Between this specific cancer and areas of high soil iodine, the relationship is r = −0.62944, p = 0.0004. This link is even clearer in non-white females, where there is

		1	2	3	4	5	6
47 Thyroid	WM	Na -0.43722 0.0019 (VL)	K -0.42342 0.0027 (VL)	Ba -0.41851 0.0031 (VL)	Zn -0.40802 0.0040 (VL)	Fe 0.40485 0.0043 (L)	-
	NWM	Zr 0.56414 0.0022 (L)	Ti 0.54899 0.0030 (L)	Ba 0.52632 0.0048 (VH)	Nb -0.52261 0.0052 (VH)	B -0.51682 0.0065 (H)	Sr 0.45200 0.0179 (H)
	WF	K -0.57507 0.0001 (VL)	Ba -0.49495 0.0003 (VL)	Na -0.48561 0.0005 (VL)	P -0.45359 0.0012 (VL)	Mn -0.45113 0.0013 (VL)	Zn 0.44392 0.0016 (VH)
	NWF	Ba 0.83272 0.0001 (VH)	Sr 0.63537 0.0004 (H)	B 0.49533 0.0086 (L)	Ga 0.48128 0.0110 (H)	Al 0.45883 0.0161 (VH)	Yb 0.45447 0.0172 (L)
48 Bone	WM	Ca -0.51821 0.0002 (VH)	Sr 0.51433 0.0002 (H)	Zr -0.45735 0.0011 (VL)	Nb 0.45356 0.0012 (M)	B -0.40882 0.0039 (L)	-
	NWM	K -0.40757 0.0348 (VH)	Se 0.40407 0.0366 (VL)	-	-	-	-
	WF	K -0.54255 0.0001 (VH)	Ca -0.54091 0.0001 (H)	Na -0.53016 0.0001 (VH)	Se -0.50158 0.0003 (VH)	Sr -0.49512 0.0003 (VH)	Ca 0.48151 0.0005 (VL)
	NWF	Na -0.61111 0.0007 (H)	Ba -0.57300 0.0018 (VH)	Ca 0.52884 0.0046 (VL)	La 0.52867 0.0046 (VH)	Nd -0.49555 0.0086 (VL)	F 0.45699 0.0166 (M)

KEY: - Letters in the upper left hand corner of each cell are the generally accepted abbreviations for elements, for example,
Se = selenium.
- WM = white males   NWM = non-white males   WF = white females   NWF = non-white females
- VL = very low   L = low   M = medium   H = high   VH = very high ── concentrations of a particular element in
surficial sediment or soils, as defined by Shacklette et al., 1971.

a marked correlation between mortality from thyroid cancer and the spatial distribution of goitre in World War I troops (r = 0.78449, p = 0.0001). The author cannot explain why potassium and sodium are not associated with thyroid cancer in non-whites, while iodine clearly appears to be. In contrast, the reverse is true of both white males and females (Table 11,2).

For white males, there is a belt of states along the Pacific coast that has decreased death rates from bone cancer, with elevated levels occurring in Kentucky, West Virginia and Pennsylvania. For white women the trends are similar.[52] It would appear from Table 11,2 that high levels of calcium, potassium and sodium are found in these low risk areas. In contrast, elevated bone cancer mortality appears to occur where there are low concentrations of these elements in surficial sediments.

Cancer of the Connective Tissue, Reticulum-Cell Sarcoma, Lymphosarcoma and Other Primary Malignant Lymphoid Neoplasms

While it is possible that elevated soil levels of sodium, potassium, barium and gallium may be associated with cancer of the connective tissue, the highest positive correlations, in the analysis, are with environmental variables (Tables 12,2 and 4,2). In non-white males and white females, the strongest correlations are with the cultivation of hay and oats. In non-white

TABLE 12,2   Cancer of Connective Tissue, Reticulum Cell Sarcoma, Lymphosarcoma, Other Lymphoid Neoplasms: Pearson Correlation Coefficients for Specific Cancers with Individual Elements

		1	2	3	4	5	6
49 Connective Tissue	WM	Ga -0.50887 0.0002 (VL)	K -0.48714 0.0004 (VL)	Ba -0.44233 0.0016 (VL)	Na -0.43447 0.0020 (VL)	Al -0.43166 0.0022 (VL)	Sr -0.43038 0.0023 (VL)
	NWM	Ba -0.52881 0.0046 (VH)	Zr -0.54745 0.0031 (VL)	-	-	-	-
	WF	Ca -0.46023 0.0010 (VL)	-	-	-	-	-
	NWF	Ga -0.45212 0.0179 (VL)	Na 0.43530 0.0232 (L)	Ba 0.42339 0.0278 (M)	Ni 0.41513 0.0313 (H)	Y 0.41988 0.0292 (L)	Mn 0.41104 0.0332 (H)
50 Reticulum Cell Sarcoma	WM	Al 0.61923 0.0006 (L)	As -0.43714 0.0019 (VH)	Fe 0.40575 0.0042 (H)	-	-	-
	NWM	Na 0.68213 0.0001 (M)	Mg 0.57878 0.0016 (VH)	Mn 0.57461 0.0017 (VH)	Zn -0.55761 0.0025 (VL)	Ca -0.55068 0.0029 (VL)	K -0.53897 0.0037 (VL)
	WF	As -0.48775 0.0004 (VH)	As 0.44348 0.0016 (VL)	Cr -0.41617 0.0033 (M)	-	-	-
	NWF	P -0.50525 0.0072 (VL)	Ca 0.50186 0.0077 (M)	Hg 0.48764 0.0099 (VH)	Li -0.48460 0.0104 (L)	P -0.45673 0.0166 (L)	K -0.43997 0.0216 (VL)
51 Lymphosarcoma	WM	Ba -0.43157 0.0022 (VL)	Pb 0.43047 0.0023 (VH)	K -0.40515 0.0043 (VL)	-	-	-
	NWM	P -0.64815 0.0003 (L)	B -0.55589 0.0026 (H)	Zn -0.54913 0.0030 (VL)	Na -0.53067 0.0044 (VL)	P -0.50267 0.0075 (VL)	K -0.47913 0.0115 (VL)
	WF	Ba -0.43733 0.0019 (VL)	K -0.42088 0.0029 (VL)	Zn 0.40554 0.0042 (VH)	Sr -0.40050 0.0048 (VL)	-	-
	NWF	Al 0.60041 0.0009 (L)	Ni 0.58311 0.0014 (M)	P 0.56860 0.0020 (VH)	Be 0.55450 0.0027 (M)	Na 0.52439 0.0050 (M)	Sr 0.49954 0.0080 (M)
52 Other Primary Malignant Lymphoid Neoplasms	WM	Sr 0.59390 0.0001 (M)	Li 0.57194 0.0001 (M)	Co 0.50936 0.0002 (H)	Fe 0.47877 0.0006 (H)	V 0.43139 0.0022 (H)	Zr 0.40180 0.0066 (L)
	NWM	Na 0.54594 0.0032 (H)	Yb 0.53910 0.0637 (L)	Ni 0.52737 0.0047 (M)	Fe 0.51538 0.0059 (L)	Pb -0.49247 0.0091 (VL)	Sr 0.48233 0.0108 (M)
	WF	Sr 0.41521 0.0033 (M)	Li 0.45865 0.0010 (M)	-	-	-	-
	NWF	Ba 0.76581 0.0001 (VH)	Sr 0.68247 0.0001 (VH)	Ca 0.49803 0.0082 (VH)	Na 0.49400 0.0088 (VH)	Sr 0.47558 0.0122 (VH)	B 0.46799 0.0138 (L)

KEY: - Letters in the upper left hand corner of each cell are the generally accepted abbreviations for elements, for example, Se = selenium.
- WM = white males   NWM = non-white males   WF = white females   NWF = non-white females
- VL = very low   L = low   M = medium   H = high   VH = very high —— concentrations of a particular element in surficial sediment or soils, as defined by Shacklette et al., 1971.

males, for example, the correlations are moderate (r = 0.58654, p = 0.0013; r = 0.48548, p = 0.0139). This suggests that, perhaps, there may be a link between agricultural chemicals and cancer of the connective tissue. It is known that at least one widely used herbicide, alachlor, causes cancer in mice and rats.[53] It is possible that others may also be carcinogens.

While there is some evidence that reticulum-cell sarcoma is associated with excesses of calcium, potassium and phosphorus in non-whites, in whites there is a noticeable relationship with arsenic. Strangely enough, low arsenic levels appear to be related to high mortality from reticulum-cell sarcoma (Table 12,2). In non-whites there is also evidence of a connection with high levels of hay cultivation (Table 4,2). This agricultural relationship is also seen for lymphosarcoma in non-white males. However, an excess of potassium, phosphorus and zinc also seem linked to this illness. The term "other primary malignant lymphoid neoplasms" is used to describe a variety of cancers including chloroma, chlorosarcoma, leukosarcoma, malignant neoplasms of any lymph gland and of the spleen. Probably, for this reason, it is very difficult to discover any consistent relationships in the data (Tables 4,2 and 12,2).

Hodgkin's Disease, Giant Follicular Lymphoma, Other Reticuloses, Mycosis Fungoides, Multiple Myeloma (Plasmocytoma) and all Lymphomas

It appears from the data presented in Table 13,2 that Hodgkin's disease is perhaps associated with high levels of soil potassium, sodium, phosphorus and strontium. Although the correlations are too low to appear on Table 13,2, elevated concentrations of zinc and mercury may also be implicated. The appearance of mercury, as a possible causal agent, when selenium is not apparently protective, is also a unique aspect of this specific cancer. In addition, the use of de-icing salt on highways may be related to mortality from this disease (Table 4,2).

There appears to be nothing of significance in the correlations between soil chemistry and giant follicular lymphoma. However, several suggestive relationships between environmental variables and this cancer are apparent. In particular, in non-white males there is a high correlation with oat (r = 0.80541, p = 0.0001) and a moderate correlation (r = 0.57708, p = 0.0016) with hay cultivation (Table 4,2).

The spatial distribution of other reticuloses, a term which includes bone marrow neoplasms and malignant reticulosis, and reticulosis or lymphoma (not otherwise specified), shows relatively poor correlations with soil element concentrations. However, it correlates positively, in white and non-white males and females, with both the cultivation of oats and the use of de-icing salts on highways. In non-white males, for example, the correlation is marked (r = 0.67207, p = 0.0002; r = 0.61157, p = 0.0015) (Table 4,2).

There is also little in the analysis to suggest that there is a relationship between soil element concentrations and mycosis fungoides (Table 13,2). However, the distribution pattern of this illness tends to correlate with indications of manufacturing activity, such as the industrial use of water, river and air pollution, toxic waste storage and the amount of strip mining activity. All of these variables suggest that there may be an association between this cancer and exposure to some industrial carcinogen(s) (Table 4,2).

TABLE 13,2 Hodgkin's Disease, Giant Follicular Lymphoma, Other Reticuloses, Mycosis Fungoides, Multiple Myeloma and All Lymphomas: Pearson Correlation Coefficients for Specific Cancers with Individual Elements

		1	2	3	4	5	6
53 Hodgkin's Disease	WM	Zr 0.60118 0.0001 (L)	Sr 0.56475 0.0001 (M)	Pb 0.50359 0.0003 (M)	P 0.48290 0.0005 (H)	P -0.43991 0.0018 (L)	Co 0.42540 0.0026 (H)
	NWM	Se 0.59023 0.0012 (M)	Na 0.59012 0.0012 (H)	As 0.58337 0.0014 (H)	K 0.57672 0.0017 (M)	Ca 0.55933 0.0024 (M)	Al 0.53641 0.0039 (VH)
	WF	Hg 0.54386 0.0001 (VH)	P 0.51199 0.0002 (L)	Ti 0.48840 0.0004 (M)	Zr 0.46439 0.0004 (M)	Mg -0.45965 0.0010 (VL)	K 0.45404 0.0012 (M)
	NWF	Sr 0.71777 0.0001 (M)	Ca -0.63635 0.0004 (VL)	P -0.60007 0.0009 (VL)	Na -0.58918 0.0012 (VL)	Na 0.58320 0.0014 (M)	Cr 0.58256 0.0014 (L)
54 Giant Follicular Lymphoma	WM	-	-	-	-	-	-
	NWM	K 0.66044 0.0002 (VH)	Na 0.63522 0.0004 (M)	Be -0.47790 0.0117 (VL)	Sr 0.45595 0.0168 (M)	Yb 0.40167 0.0378 (L)	-
	WF	Nd 0.41704 0.0032 (VL)	-	-	-	-	-
	NWF	Mo 0.54168 0.0035 (VH)	Mo -0.54168 0.0035 (VL)	Hg 0.52748 0.0047 (M)	Al 0.49138 0.0092 (VH)	Nd 0.44624 0.0196 (M)	Co 0.41664 0.0306 (VH)
55 Other Reticuloses	WM	Ga 0.40091 0.0047 (L)					
	NWM	Na 0.59143 0.0012 (H)	Zr 0.55725 0.0025 (L)	Ga 0.54647 0.0032 (L)	Mn 0.53566 0.0040 (L)	K 0.53239 0.0043 (M)	Na -0.52548 0.0049 (VL)
	WF	Hg 0.44180 0.0017 (VH)	Nb -0.41229 0.0036 (VH)	K 0.41057 0.0037 (M)	-	-	-
	NWF	Ba 0.49714 0.0083 (VH)	Ni -0.42670 0.0264 (H)	-	-		
56 Mycosis Fungoides	WM	-	-	-	=		
	NWM	Be -0.55026 0.0030 (VL)	Na 0.53596 0.0040 (L)	Ti -0.48519 0.0103 (M)	Yb -0.48095 0.0111 (M)	Li -0.47363 0.0126 (M)	Fe -0.43064 0.0249 (M)
	WF	Mo -0.50180 0.0003 (VL)					
	NWF	Na 0.66985 0.0001 (H)	Co 0.56242 0.0023 (H)	Se 0.53366 0.0042 (M)	K 0.52642 0.0048 (M)	B 0.49064 0.0094 (VL)	Pb 0.44907 0.0188 (VL)
57 Multiple Myeloma (Plasmocytoma)	WM	Ca -0.42410 0.0027 (VL)	B 0.41062 0.0010 (L)	Nb -0.40826 0.0040 (VH)	La -0.40150 0.0047 (VH)	-	-
	NWM	Sr 0.65631 0.0002 (M)	K -0.60704 0.0008 (VL)	Na -0.59062 0.0012 (VL)	P -0.58898 0.0012 (VL)	Zn -0.58504 0.0014 (VL)	Ca 0.57079 0.0019 (M)
	WF	La 0.43100 0.0022 (VL)	-	-	-	-	-
	NWF	Mg -0.71819 0.0001 (VL)	P -0.70555 0.0001 (VL)	K -0.63740 0.0004 (VL)	Ga -0.62570 0.0005 (VL)	Sr -0.61328 0.0007 (VL)	Zr -0.57867 0.0016 (VH)
58 All Lymphomas	WM	Ca -0.53396 0.0001 (VL)	Sr -0.52653 0.0001 (VL)	Mg -0.52388 0.0001 (VL)	Zr -0.52233 0.0001 (VH)	Na -0.52012 0.0002 (VL)	K -0.48026 0.0006 (VL)
	NWM	Zn 0.60478 0.0008 (VL)	Na -0.60473 0.0008 (VL)	K -0.60358 0.0008 (VL)	P -0.59821 0.0010 (VL)	Fe 0.58742 0.0013 (L)	K 0.57726 0.0016 (M)
	WF	Ca -0.54600 0.0001 (VL)	Na -0.52209 0.0001 (VL)	Mg -0.51531 0.0002 (VL)	Sr -0.51836 0.0002 (VL)	K 0.49938 0.0003 (M)	Nb -0.49099 0.0004 (VH)
	NWF	P -0.79726 0.0001 (VL)	K -0.75591 0.0001 (VL)	Sr -0.72924 0.0001 (VL)	Mg -0.71551 0.0001 (VL)	Na -0.71206 0.0001 (VL)	Zn -0.67822 0.0001 (VL)

KEY: - Letters in the upper left hand corner of each cell are the generally accepted abbreviations for elements, for example, "
Se = selenium.
- WM = white males   NWM = non-white males   WF = white females   NWF = non-white females
- VL = very low   L = low   M = medium   H = high   VH = very high ── concentrations of a particular element in surficial sediment or soils, as defined by Shacklette et al., 1971.

Multiple myeloma appears to be associated with an excess of potassium, sodium, zinc, phosphorus, magnesium and strontium in non-whites, but not in white males or females. However, when all lymphomas are examined as a unit, they seem to be connected with elevated exposure to a variety of bulk and soil trace elements, including calcium, strontium, sodium, magnesium, potassium, phosphorus, zinc and manganese. Although selenium appears to be of minor importance, high levels of zirconium and niobium are negatively correlated with these cancers (Table 13,2).

Lymphatic Leukemia, Myeloid Leukemia, Monocytic Leukemia, Acute Leukemia, Other and Unspecified Leukemia and All Leukemia

The attempts to discover links between various types of leukemia and soil element concentrations uncovered few meaningful relationships (Table 14,2). However, in non-white males, there appeared to be an association with elevated soil potassium, phosphorus, sodium, strontium, manganese and barium. Such links did not occur in other racial or sexual groups.

In contrast, several environmental variables correlated significantly with the distribution of this group of illnesses. In particular, there seems to be an association between the cultivation of cotton, hay and oats and the spatial distribution of leukemias as a whole. In non-white males the marked negative correlation (r = -0.72411, p = 0.0001) which occurs between leukemias and precipitation may indicate that the problem is not one of water pollution, but possibly of contamination from wind-blown dust or sprays. The analysis, however, provided no evidence of a meaningful association between leukemia and the use of nitrates or phosphate fertilizers, or with the presence of dieldrin and lindane in surface waters (Table 4,2). It seems most likely from the crops involved, therefore, that the major causal agent is some form of herbicide(s) or, less likely, pesticide(s).

Major differences were noted between specific leukemias. Lymphatic leukemia, for example, seems to be related to high strontium and elevated fluorine levels in the soil. These relationships are most obvious in white males and females and non-white males (Table 14,2). Barium is also associated with lymphatic leukemia in all four groups of individuals. Nevertheless, there are significant correlations between lymphatic leukemia and a number of agricultural variables, particularly the cultivation of cotton, wheat, oats and barley (Table 4,2).

70

		1	2	3	4	5	6
59 Lymphatic Leukemia	WM	B 0.55245 0.0001 (L)	Sr 0.51862 0.0002 (H)	Ba 0.51316 0.0002 (H)	F 0.48605 0.0005 (H)	-	-
	NWM	Zn 0.67191 0.0001 (H)	Sr 0.66590 0.0001 (M)	Mn 0.61970 0.0006 (H)	Li 0.54798 0.0031 (H)	P -0.52991 0.0045 (VL)	K -0.52747 0.0047 (VL)
	WF	Sr 0.50657 0.0002 (H)	F 0.50429 0.0003 (H)	Ba 0.49312 0.0004 (H)	Pb 0.46437 0.0009 (L)	B 0.42200 0.0028 (M)	Zr 0.41071 0.0037 (M)
	NWF	Ba -0.62206 0.0005 (VH)	Hg -0.45964 0.0159 (L)	B -0.45221 0.0179 (L)	Zr -0.41403 0.0318 (VL)	-	-
60 Myeloid Leukemia	WM	Co 0.50366 0.0003 (L)	Hg -0.47381 0.0007 (H)	Cr 0.46334 0.0009 (L)	Sr 0.45207 0.0013 (H)	Sc 0.43185 0.0022 (L)	Mg 0.42169 0.0028 (L)
	NWM	Pb 0.52573 0.0049 (VH)	Ba 0.45312 0.0174 (VH)	Ba 0.40148 0.0379 (M)	-	-	-
	WF	-	-	-	-	-	-
	NWF	Pb -0.49100 0.0092 (M)	Be 0.48873 0.0097 (VH)	Ba 0.44773 0.0192 (VH)	-	-	-
61 Monocytic Leukemia	WM	Mo 0.47870 0.0006 (VH)	-	-	-	-	-
	NWM	Mo 0.56327 0.0022 (VH)	Mo -0.56327 0.0022 (VL)	Ba -0.54243 0.0035 (VH)	Mn 0.52627 0.0048 (H)	Li 0.50492 0.0072 (H)	As 0.49876 0.0081 (VL)
	WF	Mo 0.47687 0.0006 (VH)	Sc 0.45779 0.0011 (VH)	Li 0.40094 0.0047 (H)	Mo -0.41537 0.0033 (VL)	-	-
	NWF	Mg 0.50119 0.0077 (H)	Ba -0.43683 0.0227 (VL)	Mo 0.41460 0.0315 (VH)	Mo -0.41460 0.0315 (VL)	Ca -0.40538 0.0359 (VL)	Ba 0.40217 0.0376 (H)
62 Acute Leukemia	WM	F -0.42219 0.0028 (H)	-	-	-	-	-
	NWM	Ba 0.67981 0.0001 (VH)	Mg 0.60498 0.0080 (H)	Mg -0.38845 0.0013 (VL)	Cu 0.55153 0.0029 (H)	K -0.52086 0.0093 (VL)	Ga -0.49934 0.0080 (VL)
	WF	Ca -0.49390 0.0004 (H)	-	-	-	-	-
	NWF	Ca 0.50985 0.0066 (M)	Ga 0.43364 0.0236 (VH)	Cr 0.42696 0.0263 (L)	Na -0.41256 0.0325 (VL)	Pb 0.40361 0.0368 (VH)	-
63 Leukemia (other and unspecified)	WM	B 0.47803 0.0006 (H)	Zn 0.42843 0.0023 (VL)	-	-	-	-
	NWM	Ba 0.64914 0.0002 (VH)	Fe -0.48165 0.0110 (L)	Cr 0.42898 0.0256 (H)	Yb 0.42253 0.0281 (L)	Sr 0.40388 0.0367 (H)	-
	WF	B 0.55156 0.0001 (H)	Na -0.52298 0.0001 (H)	Sr -0.52003 0.0002 (VH)	Mn 0.43482 0.0020 (L)	-	-
	NWF	Se 0.50921 0.0067 (VL)	Mo -0.48899 0.0096 (VH)	Mo 0.48899 0.0096 (VL)	Cr -0.43086 0.0249 (L)	-	-
64 All Leukemia	WM	Sr 0.51625 0.0002 (H)	Ba 0.45826 0.0011 (H)	B 0.43769 0.0019 (L)	-	-	-
	NWM	K -0.72559 0.0001 (VL)	P -0.70279 0.0001 (VL)	Na -0.68102 0.0001 (VL)	Sr -0.67933 0.0001 (VL)	Mn -0.67602 0.0001 (VL)	Ba -0.65818 0.0002 (VL)
	WF	Li -0.42542 0.0026 (VH)	-	-	-	-	-
	NWF	Ba -0.59408 0.0011 (VH)	Nb -0.44053 0.0215 (L)	-	-	-	-
65 Other Unspecified Sites and Secondary Neoplasms	WM	Sr -0.58251 0.0001 (H)	Hg -0.50049 0.0003 (L)	Ca -0.43992 0.0018 (VH)	-	-	-
	NWM	V 0.42409 0.0275 (VH)	Cr 0.41824 0.0299 (VH)	Ni 0.41138 0.0330 (VH)	-	-	-
	WF	Sr -0.49430 0.0004 (H)	Hg -0.40996 0.0038 (L)	-	-	-	-
	NWF	Ba 0.53674 0.0039 (VH)	Nb 0.51726 0.0057 (L)	Mn 0.42319 0.0278 (L)	Yb -0.42235 0.0282 (VH)	Ga -0.40350 0.0369 (VH)	-
66 All Malignant Neoplasms	WM	Hg 0.58946 0.0001 (VH)	Se -0.52248 0.0001 (H)	Mg -0.48647 0.0005 (VL)	Ni -0.48501 0.0005 (H)	Be -0.46809 0.0008 (VL)	Ca -0.46634 0.0008 (VH)
	NWM	P -0.71145 0.0001 (VL)	K -0.69923 0.0001 (VL)	Mg -0.66398 0.0002 (VL)	P -0.64201 0.0003 (L)	Se -0.64695 0.0003 (H)	Hg -0.61791 0.0006 (VL)
	WF	Se -0.59331 0.0001 (H)	Be -0.56671 0.0001 (VL)	Hg -0.53971 0.0001 (VL)	P -0.52587 0.0001 (L)	P -0.52107 0.0001 (VL)	Mn -0.51874 0.0002 (VL)
	NWF	P -0.78520 0.0001 (VL)	K -0.77845 0.0001 (VL)	Sr -0.65766 0.0002 (VL)	Ba -0.65115 0.0002 (VL)	Mn -0.63687 0.0004 (VL)	Na -0.59890 0.0010 (VL)

KEY: - Letters in the upper left hand corner of each cell are the generally accepted abbreviations for elements, for example,
- WM = white males   NWM = non-white males   NWF = non-white females
- VL = very low   L = low   M = medium   H = high   VH = very high — concentrations of a given element in
surficial sediment or soils, as defined by Shacklette et al., 1971.

There are no obvious relationships between myeloid leukemia and soil element concentrations, although there is some evidence that high levels of barium may be associated with this illness in non-whites. However, most of the more consistent relationships appear to be with agricultural production, especially the growth of wheat, oats and hay (Table 4,2). Since nitrates or phosphates are not involved, this illness does not appear to be related to fertilizer use.

Monocytic leukemia, in contrast, seems to be associated, in part, to very high levels of molybdenum in soils. In non-white males, for example, the relationship is moderate ($r = 0.56327$, $p = 0.0022$). Strangely enough, this disease also correlates negatively with the growth of tobacco in all four groups. Its highest association is a marked correlation found in non-white females ($r = -0.60860$, $p = 0.0161$). The reason for this negative correlation is unknown, but it should be noted that tobacco is almost invariably grown on sandy, well drained soils that are likely to be low in heavy metals.

Given the apparent relationship between agriculture and lymphatic, myeloid and monocytic leukemias, it is to be expected that these cancers would be elevated in farming areas. In the United States, lymphatic leukemia displays increased death rates in the central and north midwest, while lowest mortality occurs in the industrial northeast. This is true for both male and female whites.[54] Monocytic leukemia tends to result in high mortality in Indiana, Michigan, Ohio, California, Hawaii and Oregon in white males. The same is true of white females, except that there is an additional peak in the central midwest. Non-white mortality peaks occur in California and Hawaii, Ohio and Michigan.[55] Clearly, mortality from leukemia is particularly elevated in farming communities. This is also true for Canada and England and Wales.

Acute leukemia, leukemia (other and unspecified), and secondary and unspecified neoplasms are all collective categories of cancer, which include a variety of specific illnesses and, therefore, correlate poorly with soil and environmental variables.

Conclusions: All Malignant Neoplasms

A final set of Pearson correlation coefficients were calculated to illustrate the strength of relationships between soil element concentrations and environmental variables and the spatial distribution of all malignant neoplasm mortalities in the United States. From the results, several conclusions can be reached. The most important natural protective element against cancer appears to be selenium. This study, for example, provides evidence that, in white males, selenium is associated with reduced mortality from at least 15 specific cancers. In particular, it appears to be beneficial in reducing the death rate from cancers of the digestive system. This is not universally true, and it will not apparently be of value in lowering mortality from cancer of the lip, salivary gland, nasopharynx, liver, pancreas or peritonium. Nevertheless, selenium appears to act as an important preventative agent against five of the ten most significant global cancers,[56] namely those of the mouth, pharynx, esophagus, colon and rectum, bladder and, to a lesser extent, the lung. Selenium is also associated with reduced mortality from cancer of the larynx. Oddly enough, while there is little evidence that it is of value against cancer of the pancreas in white males, it appears protective in non-whites. In women, it also seems to be of value in lowering mortality from cancer in certain sexual organs, namely those of the ovary, uterus and breast. However, the evidence for a protective role against breast cancer is stronger in non-white women than in whites. Conversely, the most dangerous natural carcinogen appears to be mercury, probably because it reduces the body's capacity to assimilate selenium.[57]

There are major differences in racial susceptibility to various elements, non-whites being particularly vulnerable to elevated levels of phosphorus, potassium, sodium, magnesium, manganese, zinc, strontium and barium in soils. Of special interest are high levels of calcium which appear generally protective in whites, but possibly even, on balance, a threat to non-whites. The differences between the sexes are less marked, in both whites and non-whites.

The major environmental variables associated with the distribution of cancer in the United States appear to be the use of de-icing salt on highways, low selenium concentrations in animal fodder, toxic waste site distribution, industrial water withdrawal uses and coal mining (Table 4,2).

These analyses also appear to indicate that sunlight may be of major importance in reducing mortality from several cancers, such as those of the large intestine, the rectum and breast cancer. It is suggested that this is probably because of its role in the production of vitamin D, which assists in the use of calcium.

Figures 10,1 and 11,1 illustrate the distribution of total cancer mortality in the United States and demonstrate that the highest levels are in the northeast, especially in Rhode Island, New York State, Maryland and the District of Columbia. In these areas, industrial carcinogens and road salt are widely dispersed, while concurrently there is relatively little calcium and selenium present in the soils. In contrast, the lowest cancer rates, in the United States, occur in New Mexico. Here there is relatively little industry or agriculture and the soils are rich in calcium, strontium, barium and magnesium. In addition, moderate soil element levels of phosphorus, potassium, sodium and zinc predominate.[58] Cancers associated with either too much, or too little, of these elements, therefore, appear relatively uncommon. However, as might be anticipated, since cancer of the biliary passages and liver appears to be associated with high levels of calcium, strontium, barium and magnesium, this disease is very common in New Mexico. The age adjusted death rates per 100,000 for the United States as a whole from this disease are 2.956, 3.691, 3.707, and 2.528 for white and non-white males, and white and non-white females, respectively. In New Mexico, the least cancer prone state in the United States, the rates are 2.775, 6.773, 4.559 and 12.273.[59]

From this discussion of the possible links between soil element concentrations and environmental variables and cancer, the reasons for high positive and negative correlations between specific cancers themselves becomes obvious (Figures 1,1 and 2,1). It may be recalled, for example, that mortality from most digestive organ and respiratory cancers had fairly similar spatial distributions. This appears to be because calcium and selenium seem to reduce mortality from both illnesses, while high levels of industrial carcinogens, road salt and potassium, phosphorus, magnesium, and sodium appear to promote it. Breast cancer and cancer of the ovary appear related through similar associations (Table 6,2). The unique distribution of the leukemias, apparently the result of agricultural pesticide or insecticide use, also becomes understandable.

These fundamental associations also appear to explain why, when a factor analysis of human cancer in the United States was attempted, Factor I alone accounted for a very unusual 60.65 percent of the variance (Figure 9,1). This is because mortality rates for many specific cancers have similar spatial distributions, the highest death rate being commonest where magnesium, manganese, phosphorus, potassium and zinc are elevated in soils and calcium and selenium levels are low.[60] In addition, these high total cancer mortality states apply excessive quantities of de-icing salt to their highways and are involved in the large scale industrial use of water and in toxic waste storage. While some of these variables may only appear in the analyses because of their chance relationships with other activities or elements, as a whole, they appear to implicate both manmade and natural pollution as the major causes of cancer.

REFERENCES

1. MAGNUSON, E., "The Problem that Cannot be Buried", *Time*, vol. 126(15), 1985, p. 71.

2. GERAGHTY, J.J., MILLER, D.W., VAN DER LEEDEN, F. and TROISE, F.L., *Water Atlas of the United States*. Port Washington, New York: Water Information Centre, 1973, 122 plates.

3. DELURY, G.E. (ed.), *The World Almanac and Book of Facts*. New York: Newspaper Enterprise Association Inc., 1975, pp. 129-135.

4. McCORMICK, R.A., "Air Pollution Climatology" in STERN, A.C. (ed.), *Air Pollution*. New York: Academic Press, 1968, pp. 275-321.

5. SHACKLETTE, H.T., HAMILTON, J.C., BOERNGEN, J.G., and BOWLES, J.M., "Elemental Composition of Surficial Materials in the Conterminous United States", *Geological Survey Professional Paper 574-D*, 1971a, 71 pp.; SHACKLETTE, H.T., BOERNGEN, J.G., CAHILL, J.P. and RAHILL, R.L., "Lithium in Surficial Materials of the Conterminous United States and Partial Data on Cadmium", *Geological Survey Circular 673*, 1973, 8 pp.; SHACKLETTE, H.T., BOERNGEN, J.G. and TURNER, R.L., "Mercury in the Environment in Surficial Materials of the Conterminous United States", *Geological Survey Circular 644*, 1971b, 5 pp.; SHACKLETTE, H.T., BOERNGEN, J.G. and KEITH, J.R., "Selenium, Fluorine and Arsenic in Surficial Materials of the Conterminous United States", *Geological Survey Circular 692*, 1974, 14 pp.

6. SHACKLETTE, *et al.*, 1971a, *op. cit.*.

7. BURBANK, F., *Patterns in Cancer Mortality in the United States: 1950-1967*. National Cancer Institute Monograph 33, United States Department of Health, Education and Welfare, 1971, 594 pp.

8. KELLER, E.A., *Environmental Geology*, 2nd Edition. Columbus: Charles Merrill, 1979, pp. 324-359.

9. KIRKPATRICK, T., "Barium Compounds", in *Encyclopedia of Chemical Technology*, 3rd Edition, vol. 3. New York: John Wiley, 1978, pp. 463-479.

10. KIRSCHMANN, J.D. and DUNNE, L.J., *Nutrition Almanac*, 2nd Edition. New York: McGraw-Hill, 1984, 313 pp.

11. HILL, C.H., "Reversal of Selenium Toxicity in Chicks by Mercury and Cadmium", *Environment Health Perspective*, vol. 4, 1973, pp. 104-105; HILL, C.H., "Interrelationship of Selenium with Other Trace Elements", *Proc. Fed American Society Experimental Biology*, vol. 34(1), 1975, pp. 2096-2100; FROSETH, J.A., PIPER, R.C. and CARLSON, J.R., "Relationship of Dietary Selenium and Oral Methylmercury to Blood and Tissue Selenium and Mercury Concentrations and Deficiency — Toxicity Signs in Swine", *Proc. Fed. American Society Experimental Biology*, vol. 33 (3, part 1), 1974, p. 660.

12. ZELLER, A.F., "Strontium and Strontium Compounds" in *Encyclopedia of Chemical Technology*, 3rd Edition, vol. 21. New York: John Wiley, 1983, pp. 762-769.

13. *Ibid.*

14. KIRSCHMANN and DUNNE, *op. cit.*, pp. 64-100.

15. *Ibid.*, pp. 12-64.

16. *Ibid.*

17. *Ibid.*

18. SUBCOMMITTEE ON SELENIUM, Committee on Animal Nutrition, Board of Agriculture, National Research Council, *Selenium in Nutrition*, Revised Edition. Washington, D.C.: National Academy Press, 1983, pp. 73-74.

19. KIRSCHMANN and DUNNE, *op. cit.*, pp. 100-108.

20. *Ibid.*

21. *Ibid.*, pp. 12-64.

22. HILL, 1973 and 1975, *op. cit.*

23. BURBANK, *op. cit.*, pp. 122-180.

24. STRAHLER, A.N. and STRAHLER, A.H., *Elements of Physical Geography*. New York: John Wiley, 1984, pp. 372-398.

25. GERAGHTY, *et al.*, *op. cit.*, plate 66, "Water Pollution from De-icing Salts".

26. MASON, J.T., McKAY, F.W., HOOVER, R., BLOT, W.J. and FRAUMENI, J.F. Jr., *Atlas of Cancer Mortality for U.S. Counties: 1950-1969*. DHEW Publication No. (NIH) 75-780, U.S. Department of Health, Education and Welfare, 1975.

27. GERAGHTY, *et al.*, *op. cit.*

28. *Ibid.*

29. YUNIS, J.J. and HOFFMAN, W.R., "Birth of an Errant Cell". *The Sciences*, Nov./Dec. 1985, pp. 29-30.

30. KIRSCHMANN and DUNNE, *op. cit.*, p. 105.

31. GLICK, B.J., "The Spatial Organization of Cancer Mortality", *Annals, Association of American Geographers*, vol. 74(4), 1982, pp. 471-481.

32. PARKIN, D.M., STJERNSWARD, J. and MUIR, C.S., "Estimates of the Worldwide Frequency of Twelve Major Cancers". *Bulletin of the World Health Organization*, vol. 62(2), 1984, pp. 163-182.

33. BURBANK, *op. cit.*, p. 240.

34. KIRSCHMANN and DUNNE, *op. cit.*, p. 105.

35. GARDNER, M.J., "Mapping Cancer Mortality in England and Wales", *British Medical Bulletin*, vol. 40(4), 1984, pp. 320-328. See also ARMSTRONG, B.K., "Melanoma of the Skin" *British Medical Journal*, vol. 40(4), 1984, pp. 346-350.

36. *Ibid.*

37. ELWOOD, J.M., LEE, J.A.H., WALTER, S.D., MO, T. and GREEN, A.E.S., "Relationship of Melanoma and Other Skin Cancer Mortality to Latitude and Ultraviolet Radiation in the United States and Canada", *International Journal of Epidemiology*, vol. 3, 1974, pp. 325-332.

38. HERRON, J., "The Geographical Distribution of Malignant Melanoma in Queensland", *Medical Journal of Australia*, vol. 2, 1969, pp. 892-894.

39. GREEN, A. and SISKIND, V., "Geographical Distribution of Cutaneous Melanoma in Queensland", *Medical Journal of Australia*, vol. 3, 1983, pp. 407-410.

40. ARMSTRONG, *op. cit.*, pp. 346-350.

41. HOLMAN, C.D.J., MULRONEY, C.D. and ARMSTRONG, B.K., "Epidemiology of Preinvasive and Invasive Malignant Melanoma in Western Australia", *International Journal of Cancer*, vol. 25, 1980, pp. 317-323.

42. BERAL, V. and ROBINSON, N., "The Relationship of Malignant Melanoma, Basal and Squamous Skin Cancers to Indoor and Outdoor Work", *British Journal of Cancer*, vol. 44, 1981, pp. 886-891.

43. MASON, *et al.*, *op. cit.*

44. BURBANK, *op. cit.*, p. 387.

45. KELLER, *op. cit.*, p. 353.

46. BURBANK, *op. cit.*, pp. 405 and 414.

47. *Ibid.*, p. 405.

48. *Ibid.*, p. 414.

49. PENDERGAST, W.J., MILMORE, B.K. and MARCUS, S.C., "Thyroid Cancer and Thyrotoxicosis in the United States: Their Relation to Endemic Goitre", *Journal of Chronic Disease*, vol. 13, 1961, pp. 22-38.

50. STRAIN, W.H., PORIES, W.J., MANSOUR, E.G. and FLYNN, A., "Therapies for Environmental Element Deficiencies and Toxic Excess", *Geological Survey of America Special Paper 155*, 1975, pp. 83-105.

51. *Ibid.*

52. BURBANK, *op. cit.*, p. 432.

53. THE CANADIAN PRESS, "Cancer-causing 'Lasso' Imported Despite Wise Ban", *Times-Colonist*, Dec. 7, 1985, p. C8.

54. BURBANK, *op. cit.*, p. 531.

55. *Ibid.*, p. 549.

56. PARKIN, *et al.*, *op. cit.*

57. HILL, 1973 and 1975, *op. cit.*

58. SHACKLETTE, *et al.*, 1971a, *op. cit.*

59. BURBANK, *op. cit.*, p. 141.

60. SHACKLETTE, *et al.*, 1971a, *op. cit.*

*Reducing the risk of death from cancer
is a major public health priority in the
United States. Cancer now represents the
second most important cause of death
[after heart disease] and, by most accounts,
is the most troubling because of its painful
history and the apparent randomness of
its victims.*

David Harrison Jr., 1981

3 THE SEARCH FOR MULTIPLE RELATIONSHIPS

METHOD OF ANALYSIS:
STEPWISE MULTIPLE REGRESSION

Multiple regression is a useful method for predicting the response of a dependent variable that is known to be influenced by the simultaneous effects of one or more independent variables.[1] Multiple regression can also be used as a research technique in identifying which combinations of many independent variables, available for testing, can best explain the observed variation in the dependent variable.[2] This application has been termed stepwise regression.[3]

The general model used is:

$$Y = \alpha + \beta_1 X_1 + \beta_2 X_2 + \ldots \beta_K X_K + \epsilon , \qquad (1)$$

where Y, the state age standardized cancer mortality rate, is a response that is, in part, linearly dependent on one or more variables, designated by X.[4] The Xs are in this case the soil and environmental variable listed in Table 1,2. However, in a few instances complete data about the concentrations of specific soil elements were only available in two or three groups, rather than the five normal classes. When this was the case, absent classes were represented by zero data in the input, to maintain the integrity of the set, but these missing groups were not retained for the final analysis. Similarly, any environmental variable for which the data was significantly incomplete was also deleted before stepwise regression was undertaken. These omissions reduced the number of soil and environmental variables, that is Xs, to 219.

The stepwise procedure used to select variables was one of the step-up variety, in the classification used by Snedecor and Cochran.[5] Each X is adjusted by a regression coefficient β . The regression constant, α , is the intercept of the regression line with the Y axis, when all of the X terms equal zero, while the variable ϵ is the portion of the age standardized mortality rate that could not be described by the regression equation.

In stepwise regression, the first variable entered is one that has the highest linear correlation with the dependent variable Y. The procedure then examines the standardized partial regression coefficients of the other independent variables and selects the variable having the highest coefficient to add to the regression equation. Each time a variable is added, all variables are tested for statistical significance at the 0.05 level. Any that are found not to account for significant reductions in the variance of Y are deleted. The procedure can be continued until all variables in the equation are significant and all those outside are not.[6] In this particular case, the author specified that only the three most important variables were to be identified. Since it is still possible that there may be links between these three X variables, care has to be taken in interpretation and in making strong claims concerning how much of the variance has been explained by the regression equation. To ensure that the relationships between specific cancers and soil and environmental variables were linear, several regression lines were plotted (Figure 1,3). These were used to visually confirm that the relationships were as anticipated.

It should also be pointed out that, ideally, there should be more observation points for the dependent variable, that is areal units, than independent variables. However, when working at the state scale this would greatly limit the number of soil and environmental variables that could be used. Again it is pointed out that the analysis, therefore, should be viewed as a means of generating hypotheses, rather than finely tuned predictive models.

White Males

With these limitations in mind, it can be seen from Table 1,3 that the stepwise regression equations for white males, on average, appear to explain some 56.4 percent of the variance. In 59.3 percent of the cases, at least 50 percent of variance can be accounted for. In 11 instances, over 70 percent appears to be explained by the impact of the three variables selected. While these results are acceptable, they are generally less impressive than those achieved with the non-white groups studied. This probably reflects the greater mobility of white males and their exposure to a wider variety of occupational carcinogens, that may not be adequately reflected in the data bank. In every case all the variables selected were statistically significant ($p > 0.05$).

Since there were 59 regression equations generated, each containing three variables, a total of 177 soil and environmental variables were identified, as being useful in predicting some type of cancer mortality, in the United States. As 219 variables were available for selection, if all were of equal significance one might have expected most to have been selected

82

Figure 1,3 Regression Lines Showing the Relationships Between Selected Cancers and Environmental Variables

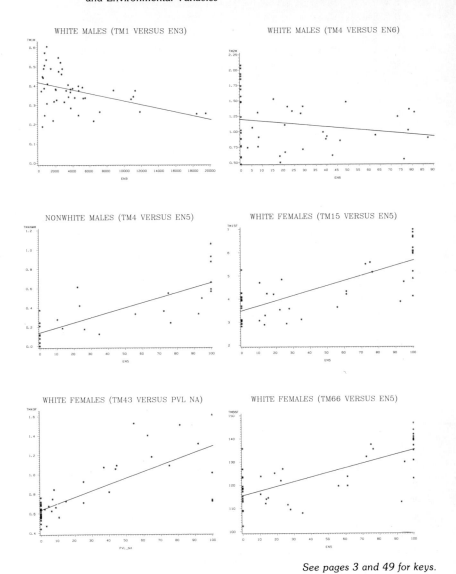

See pages 3 and 49 for keys.

Table 1,3 Stepwise Multiple Regression Equations — White Males

Dependent Variable	Three Most Significant Independent Variables (0.05 probability level)	Percentage of Total Sum of Squares of Dependent Variable Explained
TM1M (Lip)	= 0.388 − 0.00000904(EN3) − 0.0108(EN9) + 0.00180(PH Ti)	45.4
TM2M (Tongue)	= 1.155 + 0.0185(EN4) − 0.00660(PH Cr) − 0.00576(PM Sc)	74.1
TM3M (Salivary gland)	= 0.527 − 0.00542(EN18) − 0.00130(PM Pb) − 0.00134 (PM Sc)	52.1
TM4M (Floor of mouth)	= 0.247 + 0.00551(EN4) − 0.00347(PH Cr) + 0.00166(PH Sc)	80.4
TM5M (Other mouth)	= 0.301 + 0.00768(EN8) + 0.00150(EN21) + 0.201(EN65)	76.0
TM6M (Oral mesopharynx)	= 0.294 + 0.000667(EN42) − 0.00200(PM Cu) + 0.00194(PH P)	74.7
TM7M (Nasopharynx)	= 0.231 + 0.00300(EN8) + 0.000899(PH Y) − 0.00155(PL Zr)	49.2
TM8M (Hypopharynx)	= 0.249 + 0.00376(EN4) + 0.00288(EN63) − 0.00368(PM As)	56.3
TM9M (Pharynx)	= 0.249 + 0.0182(EN8) + 0.00131(EN33) + 0.00712(PL Ni)	72.9
TM10M (Buccal cavity and pharynx)	= 5.398 + 0.383(EN4) − 0.0320(PVH Ca) − 0.0254(PH Cr)	75.8

Table 1,3 (continued)

Dependent Variable	Three Most Significant Independent Variables (0.05 probability level)	Percentage of Total Sum of Squares of Dependent Variable Explained
TM11M (Esophagus)	$= 2.371 + 0.0000898(EN3) + 0.181(EN9) + 0.0859(EN65)$	73.4
TM12M (Stomach)	$= 13.946 - 0.0529(PVL\ K) + 0.0423(PM\ Na) + 0.0394(PVH\ Hg)$	67.9
TM13M (Small intestine)	$= 0.343 + 0.00562(EN65) + 0.00194(PL\ Nb) + 0.00124(PM\ K)$	45.3
TM14M (Large intestine)	$= 8.300 + 0.394(EN48) + 0.536(EN65) + 0.0462(PH\ Y)$	80.5
TM15M (Rectum)	$= 5.514 + 0.0368(EN4) + 0.0277(EN5) - 0.0298(PVL\ Na)$	79.0
TM16M (Liver)	$= 2.515 + 0.0000542(EN3) - 0.00946(PVH\ Cu) + 0.00895(PL\ Pb)$	43.2
TM17M (Pancreas)	$= 9.414 - 0.0265(PH\ Cr) + 0.0182(PH\ Fe) - 0.0185(PH\ Mn)$	43.1
TM18M (Peritoneum)	$= 0.353 + 0.667(EN53) + 0.00146(PM\ Nd) + 0.00146(PM\ Sr)$	46.4
TM19M (Digestive, unspecified)	$= 0.424 + 0.00369(EN4) - 0.00558(EN28) + 0.00241(PVH\ As)$	47.6
TM20M (All digestive)	$= 49.775 + 0.988(EN9) + 0.772(EN65) - 0.125(PVL\ K)$	72.5

Table 1,3 (continued)

Dependent Variable	Three Most Significant Independent Variables (0.05 probability level)	Percentage of Total Sum of Squares of Dependent Variable Explained
TM21M (Nose, middle ear, sinuses)	$= 0.444 + 0.00227(\text{PM Fe}) + 0.00166(\text{PL As}) - 0.00248(\text{PH Fl})$	39.8
TM22M (Larynx)	$= 1.607 + 0.00457(\text{EN21}) + 0.00316(\text{EN42}) - 0.0113(\text{PM Zn})$	72.4
TM23M (Bronchus, trachea, lung)	$= 17.183 + 0.000303(\text{EN3}) - 0.0583(\text{PM P}) - 0.0811(\text{PM Na})$	47.8
TM24M (Lung, unspecified)	$= 21.606 + 0.666(\text{EN9}) - 0.0212(\text{EN24}) - 0.120(\text{PL Hg})$	52.4
TM25M (Mediastinum)	$= 0.235 - 0.00183(\text{PH Cr}) + 0.00182(\text{PVH La}) + 0.00104(\text{PL Sr})$	32.9
TM26M (All respiratory)	$= 39.349 - 0.0263(\text{EN23}) + 0.0159(\text{EN42}) - 0.141(\text{PM Al})$	55.5
TM27M (Breast)	$= 0.251 + 0.000446(\text{EN57}) + 0.00115(\text{PM Sr}) - 0.00152(\text{PVH Zr})$	40.9
TM35M (Prostate)	$= 18.451 - 0.559(\text{EN43}) + 0.0323(\text{PH Sr}) - 0.419(\text{PL Se})$	49.9
TM36M (Testes)	$= 0.669 + 0.0710(\text{EN19}) + 0.00140(\text{PVH Co}) - 0.00192(\text{PVL Mn})$	51.9
TM37M (Male genitals, unspecified)	$= 0.347 - 0.00880(\text{EN40}) + 0.000985(\text{PVH Ga}) - 0.00148(\text{PM F})$	41.4

Table 4.3 (continued)

Dependent Variable	Three Most Significant Independent Variables (0.05 probability level)	Percentage of Total Sum of Squares of Dependent Variable Explained
TM38M (All male genitals)	$= 19.053 - 0.367(EN43) - 0.0367(PM\ Cr) + 0.457(PL\ Zr)$	47.8
TM39M (Kidney)	$= 5.509 - 0.00415(EN15) - 0.00749(PVL\ Na) - 0.0130(PH\ Hg)$	65.8
TM40M (Bladder and urinary organs)	$= 6.175 + 0.177(EN5) - 0.0174(PVL\ Mg) - 0.0286(PH\ Ni)$	65.3
TM41M (All urinary tract)	$= 10.493 + 0.228(EN5) - 0.0294(PVL\ Na) - 0.0369(PH\ F)$	69.8
TM42M (Melanoma)	$= 0.302 + 0.000800(EN11) + 0.00360(EN15) - 0.00222(EN23)$	69.3
TM43M (Skin)	$= 1.716 - 0.179(EN19) + 0.0440(EN47) + 0.119(PVH\ Zr)$	75.1
TM44M (Entire Integument)	$= 3.210 - 0.258(EN19) + 0.577(EN47) + 0.00939(PVL\ Na)$	73.0
TM45M (Eye)	$= 0.179 + 0.00299(EN47) + 0.000778(PVL\ Zn) + 0.00159(PL\ Se)$	51.1
TM46M (Nervous System)	$= 4.249 - 0.0205(PVH\ Ba) + 0.0114(PVH\ Se) - 0.00533(PVH\ Li)$	39.6
TM47M (Thyroid)	$= 0.325 + 0.0120(EN22) - 0.132(EN26) + 0.000168(EN42)$	41.9

Table 1.3 (continued)

Dependent Variable	Three Most Significant Independent Variables (0.05 probability level)	Percentage of Total Sum of Squares of Dependent Variable Explained
TM48M (Bone)	$= 1.329 - 0.00580(\text{PVH Ca}) + 0.00290(\text{PM Sr}) + 0.00319(\text{PVH Li})$	46.8
TM49M (Connective tissue)	$= 0.674 - 0.00270(\text{EN54B}) - 0.00149(\text{PVL Pb}) - 0.00153(\text{PVH Y})$	55.6
TM50M (Reticulum cell sarcoma)	$= 0.859 - 0.00215(\text{EN6}) - 0.00543(\text{PVL Fe}) + 0.00747(\text{PVL As})$	50.6
TM51M (Lymphosarcoma)	$= 2.197 + 0.0000355(\text{EN3}) + 0.00729(\text{PH Cu}) - 0.0104(\text{PL Li})$	43.6
TM52M (Other lymphoid neoplasms)	$= 0.274 + 0.000892(\text{EN33}) + 0.00609(\text{PL Li}) + 0.00831(\text{PM Li})$	55.9
TM53M (Hodgkin's disease)	$= 2.840 - 0.00204(\text{EN15}) + 0.00311(\text{PH P}) + 0.00601(\text{PL Zr})$	63.6
TM54M (Giant follicular lymphoma)	$= 0.156 + 0.0109(\text{EN13}) - 0.000240(\text{EN15}) - 0.000366(\text{PVL Ca})$	45.4
TM55M (Other reticuloses)	$= 1.0727 - 0.00137(\text{EN15}) + 0.00914(\text{PL Ga}) - 0.00592(\text{PL V})$	52.5
TM56M (Mycosis fungoides)	$= 0.0548 + 0.0000558(\text{EN42}) - 0.000376(\text{PL Nb}) - 0.000388(\text{PVH Yb})$	41.5
TM57M (Multiple myeloma)	$= 1.580 + 0.00412(\text{PVH Cr}) - 0.00386(\text{PVH La}) + 0.00448(\text{PH Sr})$	51.0

88

Table 1.3 (continued)

Dependent Variable	Three Most Significant Independent Variables (0.05 probability level)	Percentage of Total Sum of Squares of Dependent Variable Explained
TM58M (All lymphomas)	$= 11.418 - 0.00660(\text{EN15}) - 0.0120(\text{PVL Ca}) - 0.0158(\text{PL P})$	64.7
TM59M (Lymphatic leukemia)	$= 2.298 + 0.0102(\text{EN54B}) + 0.210(\text{PL B}) + 0.00853(\text{PH Zn})$	55.9
TM60M (Myeloid leukemia)	$= 1.667 + 0.00548(\text{PL Cr}) + 0.00426(\text{PM F}) - 0.00650(\text{PH Hg})$	48.4
TM61M (Monocytic leukemia)	$= 0.812 - 0.00304(\text{EN25}) + 0.00905(\text{PVH Mo}) - 0.00533(\text{PL Nb})$	46.2
TM62M (Acute leukemia)	$= 2.408 + 0.0634(\text{EN43}) + 0.00734(\text{PL Cr}) - 0.00765(\text{PH F})$	50.2
TM63M (Other leukemia)	$= 0.776 + 0.00443(\text{PH La}) + 0.00657(\text{PL Mn}) + 0.00309(\text{PVL Zn})$	46.5
TM64M (All leukemia)	$= 7.799 + 0.422(\text{EN47}) + 0.0641(\text{EN48}) + 0.0139(\text{PH Sr})$	52.2
TM65M (Other and secondary neoplasms)	$= 14.366 - 0.0136(\text{EN24}) - 0.0712(\text{PVH Sc}) - 0.0518(\text{PL Hg})$	48.0
TM66M (All malignant neoplasms)	$= 151.835 + 0.666(\text{EN4}) - 0.455(\text{PH Cr}) + 0.362(\text{PH Sc})$	69.4

See page 49 for key to environmental variables.

only once by the stepwise regression procedure. It can be seen from Table 1,3 that this was clearly not the case. Certain variables appear repeatedly, while many others are never selected. It was decided, therefore, to arbitrarily examine all variables that were selected three times or more by the procedure. While some of these variables may have simply appeared by chance, it was anticipated that others were likely to be of real importance. The author is fully aware that the use of three as a cut-off point does not imply statistical significance.

Amongst the environmental variables that appear at least three times in the equations are the total number of inhabitants and density of population of the state, the concentration of de-icing salt used on highways, industrial water use and toxic waste site density. All of these variables seem to be indicators of exposure to industrial and commercial carcinogens. Certain agricultural variables also tend to recur in the stepwise regression equations, namely the percentage of irrigated acreage and the proportion of land used to grow cotton. Both of these variables can also be interpreted as indicators of the degree and frequency of exposure to chemical carcinogens. A third group of variables, low selenium content in fodder crops, total precipitation and sunlight also reappear regularly. The significance of selenium as an inhibitor of cancer has already been discussed in some detail. Low precipitation tends to reduce the areal extent of river and groundwater pollution, while the role of sunlight, through its impact on vitamin D and on the skin, is reviewed elsewhere.

It is suggested, therefore, that most of the variables that are repeatedly selected by the stepwise regression procedure either reflect direct exposure of white males to industrial or agricultural carcinogens, or influence their diffusion and hence distribution. Since selenium appears to be a major cancer inhibitor, low levels in fodder crops probably indicate selenium deficient diets amongst local inhabitants.

Soil element levels that were selected at least three times by the stepwise regression procedure were high chromium, which recurs most frequently, very low sodium and high and medium levels of strontium. Chromium compounds are accepted as cancer causing agents,[7] possibly because they can depress the function of enzymes involved in the metabolism of organic carcinogens. This author has already demonstrated repeatedly that sodium and strontium, above certain critical levels, appear to be associated with elevated cancer mortality. In conclusion, therefore, as might have been expected, the distribution of cancer amongst white males in the United States appears to reflect their exposure to industrial, agricultural and naturally occurring carcinogens and the amount of selenium they consume.

90

Non-white Males

The stepwise multiple regression equations, generated for non-white males, were able to account for over 50 percent of the variance (Table 2,3) some 98 percent of the time. Indeed, the average variance explained was 75.2 percent, while over 80 percent could be accounted for in 17 specific or group cancers. It should be pointed out, however, that because of the problem of uneven non-white population distribution, spatial patterns of cancer mortality in only 27 states were being analyzed. Nevertheless, the predictive models appear effective.

Many of the environmental variables that repeatedly appeared in the non-white male regressions were those that had been featured in white male equations. Variables that occurred on three or more occasions included industrial water use and the amount of the state devoted to coal mining. Both of these environmental indicators probably reflect the impact of industrial carcinogens. Agricultural carcinogens were apparently represented by the repeated selection of cotton and hay cultivation, which also appear regularly in the stepwise regression equations.

The remaining five repeating environmental variables all reflected imbalances in exposure to bulk or trace elements. These were low selenium in fodder, the amount of de-icing salt used on highways, the sodium content of drinking water, the percentage of water that was fluorinated and the iodine content of the soil (as indicated by goitre in World War I troops).

Five of the six soil elements that appeared three or more times in the regression equations were also either bulk or trace elements, or their antagonists. The most prominent of these soil elements was very high barium, the known potassium antagonist. This reappeared in seven equations. Other soil elements that featured prominently were very low calcium, very high manganese, very low potassium and very high levels of zinc. Medium levels of strontium also recurred three times.

The only unanticipated element repeating in the stepwise regression equations was high lanthanum, which appeared four times. Lanthanum is a rare earth and is found as part of a mixture of elements in rocks such as basalts, granites and shales.[8] While the rare earths, including lanthanum, are considered only slightly toxic, they are commonly associated with compounds of beryllium, uranium and thorium, all of which are extremely toxic. The toxicity of rare earths on humans appears to vary with the manner in which they are introduced, being more dangerous if inhaled or injected. They are known to collect in the liver, spleen and kidney.[9] By far the worst reactions are obtained by intraperitoneal or intravenous injections. The symptoms of such extreme toxicity include writhing, atoxia, labored respiration, walking on the toes with arched back, and sedation. Central lobular necrosis of the liver also occurs, as does decreased blood pressure and possibly hyperglycemia.[10]

Table 2,3 Stepwise Multiple Regression Equations — Non-White Males

Dependent Variable	Three Most Significant Independent Variables (0.05 probability level)	Percentage of Total Sum of Squares of Dependent Variable Explained
TM1NWM (Lip)	= 0.661 − 0.00145(EN15) + 0.0217(PVH Ba) − 0.00253(PVH Zn)	79.8
TM2NWM (Tongue)	= 1.0842 − 0.0601(EN47) + 0.0131(PVH B) + 0.0180(PL V)	66.6
TM3NWM (Salivary gland)	= 0.399 − 0.0190(EN18) + 0.00307(PM P) − 0.00429(PM Sc)	67.8
TM4NWM (Floor of mouth)	= 0.187 + 0.00366(EN5) + 0.00498(PVH Mn) − 0.00570(PL Li)	82.2
TM5NWM (Other mouth)	= 1.450 − 0.0398(EN18) − 0.0248(EN47) − 0.00662(PVL Be)	78.4
TM6NWM (Oral mesopharynx)	= 0.0823 + 0.00214(EN42) − 0.00910(PM Be) + 0.0111(PM Mg)	83.7
TM7NWM (Nasopharynx)	= 0.137 + 0.0555(EN48) + 0.176(PVH P) − 0.00785(PVH Zn)	85.6
TM8NWM (Hypopharynx)	= 0.0960 + 0.0365(EN65) − 0.00385(PM Co) + 0.00432(PH Sc)	85.0
TM9NWM (Pharynx)	= 1.110 + 0.111(PVH Cr) + 0.0103(PM Sr) − 0.00545(PH Y)	44.4
TM10NWM (Buccal cavity and pharynx)	= 2.599 + 0.0264(EN5) + 0.0377(PVH Mn) + 0.0267(PVH Yb)	72.5

Table 2,3 (continued)

Dependent Variable	Three Most Significant Independent Variables (0.05 probability level)	Percentage of Total Sum of Squares of Dependent Variable Explained
TM11NWM (Esophagus)	$= 0.791 + 0.102(EN14) + 0.0176(EN42) + 0.0478(PVH\ P)$	88.8
TM12NWM (Stomach)	$= 27.452 + 0.122(PVH\ Cu) - 0.144(PH\ Se) - 0.120(PH\ Hg)$	73.3
TM13NWM (Small intestine)	$= 0.398 - 0.00190(EN7) + 0.00335(PL\ Na) - 0.00299(PVL\ Zr)$	69.0
TM14NWM (Large intestine)	$= 11.172 + 0.0436(EN14) + 6.864(EN39) - 0.0691(PVL\ K)$	70.8
TM15NWM (Rectum)	$= 5.968 + 0.00739(EN42) - 0.0343(PM\ Cu) - 0.0414(PVL\ Mn)$	82.4
TM16NWM (Liver)	$= 2.656 - 0.0315(PL\ Cu) + 0.0685(PVH\ Mg) - 0.0390(PL\ Sc)$	72.7
TM17NWM (Pancreas)	$= 13.202 - 0.0180(EN7) - 0.0429(PH\ Pb) - 0.0607(PVL\ Sr)$	80.5
TM18NWM (Peritoneum)	$= 0.471 + 0.000169(EN3) - 0.00677(PH\ La) - 0.00473(PM\ Pb)$	74.4
TM19NWM (Digestive, unspecified)	$= 0.539 + 0.0129(EN54B) + 0.00887(PL\ Nb) + 0.0125(PL\ K)$	58.6
TM20NWM (All digestive)	$= 57.553 + 0.0553(EN42) - 0.182(PVL\ Ca) + 0.218(PH\ Sc)$	89.7

Table 2,3 (continued)

Dependent Variable	Three Most Significant Independent Variables (0.05 probability level)	Percentage of Total Sum of Squares of Dependent Variable Explained
TM21NWM (Nose, middle ear, sinuses)	$= 0.749 + 0.0367(\text{PVH Ba}) - 0.00359(\text{PVH Ga}) - 0.0154(\text{PL Pb})$	72.1
TM22NWM (Larynx)	$= 1.578 + 0.0350(\text{PVH B}) - 0.0356(\text{PM Cu}) + 0.0227(\text{PL Sr})$	74.4
TM23NWM (Bronchus, trachea, lung)	$= 4.417 + 0.000486(\text{EN3}) + 0.0189(\text{EN11}) + 0.855(\text{EN48})$	78.5
TM24NWM (Lung, unspecified)	$= 14.350 + 1.335(\text{EN9}) + 2.116(\text{EN10}) - 0.509(\text{EN47})$	78.8
TM25NWM (Mediastinum)	$= 0.258 - 0.0124(\text{EN18}) + 0.00334(\text{PM Pb}) - 0.00340(\text{PM Li})$	81.1
TM26NWM (All respiratory)	$= 34.137 + 0.148(\text{EN5}) + 0.0177(\text{EN31}) - 0.155(\text{PVL K})$	79.9
TM27NWM (Breast)	$= 0.296 + 0.00326(\text{PM Nd}) - 0.00341(\text{PM Yb}) + 0.00262(\text{PM Se})$	73.3
TM35NWM (Prostate)	$= 26.127 + 0.0926(\text{EN14}) - 0.560(\text{PVH Ba}) - 0.131(\text{PL Hg})$	84.6
TM36NWM (Testes)	$= 0.224 + 0.785(\text{PVH Ba}) + 0.00724(\text{PH Na}) - 0.0163(\text{PVH Na})$	91.3
TM37NWM (Male genitals, unspecified)	$= 0.304 + 0.00741(\text{PVH B}) + 0.0106(\text{PVL Mn}) + 0.00836(\text{PM Y})$	76.8

94

Table 2.3 (continued)

Dependent Variable	Three Most Significant Independent Variables (0.05 probability level)	Percentage of Total Sum of Squares of Dependent Variable Explained
TM38NWM (All male genitals)	$= 27.162 + 0.0957(EN14) - 0.494(PVH\ Ba) - 0.131(PL\ Hg)$	81.9
TM39NWM (Kidney)	$= 2.275 + 0.183(EN18) + 0.0275(PM\ Sr) - 0.0298(PH\ Hg)$	82.9
TM40NWM (Bladder and urinary organs)	$= 3.122 + 0.0233(EN5) + 0.0272(PM\ Fe) + 0.0233(PM\ Zr)$	75.2
TM41NWM (All urinary tract)	$= 10.702 - 0.933(EN10) - 0.0550(PVL\ Sr) + 0.0684(PVL\ Ti)$	75.7
TM42NWM (Melanoma)	$= 0.415 + 0.0301(EN9) - 0.00195(EN12) - 0.0207(EN48)$	81.7
TM43NWM (Skin)	$= 1.00547 + 0.000873(EN31) - 0.01673(EN48) - 0.0116(PH\ Li)$	75.3
TM44NWM (Entire integument)	$= 1.398 + 0.000552(EN31) - 0.00815(PH\ La) - 0.00554(PM\ K)$	62.1
TM45NWM (Eye)	$= 0.0262 + 0.00334(EN47) + 0.00137(PH\ Se) - 0.00452(PL\ Fl)$	69.9
TM46NWM (Nervous system)	$= 1.949 + 0.117(EN18) + 0.0156(PL\ Cr) - 0.0131(PL\ As)$	88.2
TM47NWM (Thyroid)	$= 0.305 + 0.0196(EN18) - 0.0047(PH\ B) + 0.00210(PM\ Yb)$	76.3

95

Table 2.3 (continued)

Dependent Variable	Three Most Significant Independent Variables (0.05 probability level)	Percentage of Total Sum of Squares of Dependent Variable Explained
TM48NWM (Bone)	$= 1.230 - 0.0485(EN40) + 0.0179(PVH\ Sr) + 0.00443(PVL\ Se)$	54.2
TM49NWM (Connective tissue)	$= 0.363 + 0.000410(EN11) - 0.0184(EN18) + 0.0317(EN48)$	75.6
TM50NWM (Reticulum cell sarcoma)	$= 0.510 - 0.01568(EN47) + 0.00666(PL\ Al) + 0.00811(PM\ Sr)$	75.7
TM51NWM (Lymphosarcoma)	$= 1.343 + 0.0511(EN48) + 0.00802(PM\ Ca) - 0.0163(PL\ P)$	76.2
TM52NWM (Other lymphoid neoplasms)	$= 0.675 + 0.0855(EN10) - 0.909(EN26) + 0.0104(PL\ Fe)$	77.5
TM53NWM (Hodgkin's disease)	$= -0.221 + 0.0296(EN16) + 0.00795(PVL\ Be) + 0.00573(PVH\ Mn)$	74.0
TM54NWM (Giant follicular lymphoma)	$= -0.0617 + 0.000997(EN25) + 0.00102(PH\ La) + 0.00438(PVH\ K)$	67.6
TM55NWM (Other reticuloses)	$= 0.708 + 0.0316(EN9) - 0.00401(EN21) + 0.00703(PH\ Na)$	72.5
TM56NWM (Mycosis fungoides)	$= 0.0455 + 0.00865(EN65) + 0.000927(PVH\ Zn) - 0.001333(PH\ As)$	63.2
TM57NWM (Multiple myeloma)	$= 2.0520 + 0.239(EN9) - 0.0165(PM\ Be) + 0.0130(PL\ Na)$	86.5

Table 2.3 (continued)

Dependent Variable	Three Most Significant Independent Variables (0.05 probability level)	Percentage of Total Sum of Squares of Dependent Variable Explained
TM58NWM (All lymphomas)	$= 5.534 - 0.350(\text{EN9}) + 0.145(\text{EN48}) + 0.0303(\text{PM Ca})$	82.4
TM59NWM (Lymphatic leukemia)	$= 1.848 - 0.0138(\text{EN12}) - 0.168(\text{EN13}) + 0.0156(\text{PH Zn})$	71.9
TM60NWM (Myeloid leukemia)	$= 1.157 + 0.000553(\text{EN31}) + 0.00830(\text{PVH Pb}) - 0.00688(\text{PVH Ni})$	52.6
TM61NWM (Monocytic leukemia)	$= 0.911 + 0.00615(\text{PH Ba}) + 0.00658(\text{PL Cu}) - 0.00861(\text{PVL Mo})$	66.3
TM62NWM (Acute leukemia)	$= 1.457 + 0.00731(\text{PL Al}) + 0.480(\text{PVH Ba}) - 0.00612(\text{PVL Mg})$	74.8
TM63NWM (Other leukemia)	$= 0.629 + 0.0438(\text{PVH Ba}) + 0.00462(\text{PH Cr}) - 0.0164(\text{PVH Na})$	72.7
TM64NWM (All leukemia)	$= 5.540 + 0.0110(\text{PVH Al}) - 0.0126(\text{PVL K}) + 0.0283(\text{PH K})$	77.0
TM65NWM (Other and secondary neoplasms)	$= 32.966 - 0.0297(\text{EN15}) - 83.885(\text{EN29}) - 0.0693(\text{PH La})$	65.6
TM66NWM (All malignant neoplasms)	$= 168.439 + 0.0543(\text{EN31}) + 0.134(\text{EN42}) - 0.560(\text{PVL Ca})$	88.1

See page 49 for key to environmental variables.

White Females

The stepwise regression equations appear quite effective in explaining the variance of the spatial distribution of cancer mortality in white women (Table 3,3). The mean variance accounted for in this way is some 55.9 percent. In 62.9 percent of the cases more than 50 percent of the variance can be explained, while in 11 instances over 70 percent appears to be accounted for by the three variables selected. Amongst the environmental variables that appear at least three times in the stepwise multiple regression equations for cancer mortality in white women are the population of the state, the number of days of high air pollution potential and the impact of coal mining. These variables seem to reflect exposure to industrial carcinogens. The area of the state devoted to cotton and hay cultivation also seems significant. A third group of variables that repeat in the analysis consists of low and medium selenium content in fodder crops and the amount of sunlight received. The significance of all of these variables has already been discussed elsewhere, although it is of interest to note that selenium appears even more important as a cancer inhibitor in white women than in white men.

White women also seem more susceptible to certain soil elements than white males. This may be because, especially during the period under analysis (1950-1967), they were less involved in the work force, and therefore travelled less often. As a result, they tended to spend more time in the local community. This greater susceptibility may also be simply, or partially, due to sexual differences.

Soil elements that appear at least three times in the stepwise regression equations include very high and very low levels of arsenic. This element is a known carcinogen in humans.[11] Also repeated in the equations are high mercury, low and very low sodium and high strontium levels. These three elements and their possible carcinogenic properties have already been discussed, as has the importance of very low potassium.

Three other elements that also repeat are high fluorine, very low boron and very high gallium. Fluorine is the most reactive element known and hazards associated with fluorides are severe, yet in small quantities such inorganic fluorine compounds are beneficial, reducing dental decay. Nevertheless, large quantities of fluorides can lead to bone fracture and even death.[12] There is little toxicological data on borates, other than borax and boric acid. There are reports, for example, that death may result from the ingestion of 15 to 30 grams of borax or 2 to 5 grams of boric acid. However, high doses have been administered during neutron capture therapy for brain tumours without severe toxic effects.[13] Gallium is chemically very similar to zinc and it is known that the toxicity of metallic gallium

Table 3.3 Stepwise Multiple Regression Equations — White Females

Dependent Variable	Three Most Significant Independent Variables (0.05 probability level)	Percentage of Total Sum of Squares of Dependent Variable Explained
TM1F (Lip)	$= 0.0161 - 0.000424(\text{EN63}) + 0.000415(\text{PH Ga}) + 0.00122(\text{PVH Zr})$	56.7
TM2F (Tongue)	$= 0.338 + 0.00153(\text{PH Cu}) + 0.00152(\text{PH Na}) - 0.00262(\text{PM Li})$	52.0
TM3F (Salivary gland)	$= 0.164 + 0.00395(\text{EN18}) + 0.00610(\text{EN47}) + 0.00102(\text{PH Zr})$	49.2
TM4F (Floor of mouth)	$= 0.0834 + 0.00134(\text{EN59}) + 0.00122(\text{PVH Na}) - 0.00101(\text{PH F})$	53.5
TM5F (Other mouth)	$= 0.127 + 0.00775(\text{EN17}) + 0.00961(\text{EN47}) + 0.00393(\text{PVL P})$	80.0
TM6F (Oral mesopharynx)	$= 0.100 - 0.000780(\text{PH La}) - 0.000572(\text{PVH Mg}) + 0.00151(\text{PVH K})$	34.4
TM7F (Nasopharynx)	$= 0.154 - 0.000952(\text{PL B}) - 0.000972(\text{PM Cr}) - 0.000751(\text{PH V})$	36.9
TM8F (Hypopharynx)	$= 0.00759 + 0.000358(\text{PVH Ga}) + 0.000991(\text{PVL F}) + 0.000534(\text{PVH F})$	46.1
TM9F (Pharynx)	$= 0.144 + 0.00200(\text{EN59}) + 0.00182(\text{PVL Na}) + 0.00178(\text{PL Zr})$	58.3

Table 3.3 (continued)

Dependent Variable	Three Most Significant Independent Variables (0.05 probability level)	Percentage of Total Sum of Squares of Dependent Variable Explained
TM10F (Buccal cavity and pharynx)	$= 1.279 + 0.00957(EN17) - 0.00480(PM\ Ga) + 0.00640(PVL\ Na)$	71.4
TM11F (Esophagus)	$= 1.126 + 0.0000171(EN3) - 0.00968(EN18) - 0.00175(EN24)$	66.4
TM12F (Stomach)	$= 7.390 + 0.254(EN4) - 0.0314(PVL\ K) + 0.0327(PL\ Yb)$	64.3
TM13F (Small intestine)	$= 0.419 - 0.00206(EN6) - 0.00328(PVL\ Al) + 0.00358(PVL\ Y)$	58.7
TM14F (Large intestine)	$= 14.707 + 0.0506(EN5) - 0.0413(PVL\ B) - 0.0305(PVL\ Na)$	80.5
TM15F (Rectum)	$= 4.147 + 0.0210(EN5) - 0.0114(PVL\ B) - 0.0142(PVL\ Na)$	81.8
TM16F (Liver)	$= 2.872 + 0.00905(EN14) + 0.00326(EN23) - 0.0113(PVL\ K)$	70.4
TM17F (Pancreas)	$= 5.461 + 0.0491(EN9) - 0.00795(PVL\ Ga) + 0.00944(PVL\ As)$	41.1
TM18F (Peritoneum)	$= 0.337 + 0.0136(EN48) - 0.00259(PH\ La) + 0.00135(PM\ Ni)$	48.8

100

Table 3.3 (continued)

Dependent Variable	Three Most Significant Independent Variables (0.05 probability level)	Percentage of Total Sum of Squares of Dependent Variable Explained
TM19F (Digestive, unspecified)	$= 0.595 - 0.00281(\text{PL Al}) - 0.00257(\text{PVL Zr}) - 0.00284(\text{PH F})$	46.7
TM20F (All digestive)	$= 38.143 + 0.0877(\text{EN5}) - 0.0643(\text{PVL B}) - 0.0824(\text{PVL Na})$	78.7
TM21F (Nose, middle ear, sinuses)	$= 0.217 - 0.00145(\text{PH Zn}) + 0.00113(\text{PL Se}) + 0.00100(\text{PH F})$	45.8
TM22F (Larynx)	$= 0.251 - 0.00153(\text{PH Sr}) - 0.00191(\text{PVL Y}) - 0.00196(\text{PVL As})$	65.8
TM23F (Bronchus, trachea, lung)	$= 1.783 + 0.00159(\text{EN11}) + 0.217(\text{EN43}) - 0.0129(\text{PH Cr})$	44.0
TM24F (Lung, unspecified)	$= 3.495 + 0.893(\text{EN9}) + 0.0269(\text{PVH Ba}) - 0.0189(\text{PH Sr})$	37.5
TM25F (Mediastinum)	$= 0.632 + 0.000452(\text{EN6}) + 0.000686(\text{PH K}) - 0.000522(\text{PVH Li})$	30.9
TM26F (All respiratory)	$= 2.346 + 0.0000729(\text{EN3}) + 0.0118(\text{EN5}) + 0.00733(\text{EN15})$	43.8
TM27F (Breast)	$= 21.427 + 0.0409(\text{EN5}) + 0.327(\text{EN48}) - 0.0529(\text{PVL Mg})$	73.5

101

Table 3.3 (continued)

Dependent Variable	Three Most Significant Independent Variables (0.05 probability level)	Percentage of Total Sum of Squares of Dependent Variable Explained
TM28F (Uterine cervix)	$= 8.892 - 0.0413(EN4) + 0.0681(EN17) - 0.0386(PH\ Sr)$	70.0
TM29F (Body of uterus)	$= 0.748 + 0.107(EN48) + 0.00705(PVL\ Cr) - 0.0101(PL\ Se)$	64.1
TM30F (Other uterus)	$= 0.0237 + 0.000392(EN6) + 0.000189(EN24) + 0.000354(PVH\ B)$	52.2
TM31F (Uterus, unspecified)	$= 5.182 + 0.00231(EN31) - 0.0363(PL\ Pb) - 0.0231(PVH\ Na)$	53.4
TM32F (Ovary)	$= 11.551 + 0.0000685(EN3) - 0.00929(EN15) - 0.0163(PVL\ Na)$	63.7
TM33F (Other female genitals)	$= 1.0395 - 0.00104(EN15) + 1.533(EN29) + 0.00123(PL\ Na)$	59.6
TM34F (All female genitals)	$= 19.637 + 38.929(EN29) + 0.00418(EN31) + 0.0300(PL\ Ca)$	59.4
TM39F (Kidney)	$= 2.995 - 0.00383(EN6) - 0.00302(EN15) + 0.00778(PH\ Sr)$	68.7
TM40F (Bladder)	$= 2.162 + 0.00691(EN5) + 0.00847(PVH\ As) - 0.0105(PH\ F)$	64.0

102

Table 3.3 (continued)

Dependent Variable	Three Most Significant Independent Variables (0.05 probability level)	Percentage of Total Sum of Squares of Dependent Variable Explained
TM41F (All urinary tract)	$= 5.774 + 0.00467(EN5) - 0.00412(EN15) - 0.00781(PM\ Cr)$	61.1
TM42F (Melanoma)	$= 1.0148 + 0.0216(EN47) + 0.00430(PVL\ K) - 0.00401(PVH\ As)$	69.7
TM43F (Skin)	$= 0.618 + 0.0238(EN47) - 0.0193(PVH\ Nd) + 0.00798(PVL\ Sr)$	80.0
TM44F (Entire Integument)	$= 1.526 + 0.0380(EN47) + 0.00608(PVL\ Na) + 0.00845(PVH\ Zr)$	83.0
TM45F (Eye)	$= 0.162 + 0.000510(EN6) + 0.00101(PL\ B) + 0.00115(PL\ Hg)$	36.7
TM46F (Nervous system)	$= 2.387 + 0.135(EN28) + 0.00350(PVH\ Mg) + 0.00904(PVL\ As)$	40.7
TM47F (Thyroid)	$= 0.648 + 0.0000101(EN3) - 0.00598(EN47) - 0.00164(PVL\ K)$	56.3
TM48F (Bone)	$= 0.699 + 0.00665(EN8) - 0.00128(EN35) - 0.00203(PVH\ Ga)$	54.5
TM49F (Connective tissue)	$= 0.450 + 0.00827(EN48) + 0.00156(PH\ Ca) - 0.000795(PVL\ Mo)$	35.4

Table 3,3 (continued)

Dependent Variable	Three Most Significant Independent Variables (0.05 probability level)	Percentage of Total Sum of Squares of Dependent Variable Explained
TM50F (Reticulum cell sarcoma)	$= 0.663 - 0.00433(\text{PVH La}) + 0.00433(\text{PM Nd}) - 0.00496(\text{PVH As})$	62.9
TM51F (Lymphosarcoma)	$= 1.720 + 0.0000224(\text{EN3}) - 0.0132(\text{EN8}) + 0.00452(\text{PL Sr})$	52.8
TM52F (Other lymphoid neoplasms)	$= 0.531 + 0.00340(\text{PM Sr}) - 0.00349(\text{PH Se}) - 0.00506(\text{PH Hg})$	43.5
TM53F (Hodgkin's disease)	$= 0.995 + 0.00459(\text{PH P}) + 0.00436(\text{PM Na}) + 0.00449(\text{PVH Hg})$	58.2
TM54F (Giant follicular lymphoma)	$= 0.0276 - 0.0000581(\text{EN31}) + 0.000360(\text{PVL Nd}) + 0.000275(\text{PM Nb})$	40.7
TM55F (Other reticuloses)	$= 0.285 - 0.00298(\text{PVH Nb}) + 0.00271(\text{PL Li}) + 0.00257(\text{PVH Hg})$	46.9
TM56F (Mycosis fungoides)	$= 0.122 + 0.000228(\text{EN6}) - 0.00102(\text{PVL Mo}) - 0.000960(\text{PVH Mo})$	59.0
TM57F (Multiple myeloma)	$= 1.0243 + 0.00299(\text{PH Ba}) + 0.00423(\text{PVL La}) - 0.00465(\text{PL As})$	46.0
TM58F (All lymphomas)	$= 7.137 - 0.00432(\text{EN15}) - 0.113(\text{PVL Ca}) + 0.00740(\text{PVH Hg})$	58.7

104

Table 3,3 (continued)

Dependent Variable	Three Most Significant Independent Variables (0.05 probability level)	Percentage of Total Sum of Squares of Dependent Variable Explained
TM59F (Lymphatic leukemia)	$= 1.443 + 0.0120(EN28) - 0.000830(EN42) + 0.00323(PM\ P)$	58.0
TM60F (Myeloid leukemia)	$= 1.0751 + 0.769(EN19) + 0.00288(PL\ Mg) - 0.00371(PVH\ Mo)$	33.8
TM61F (Monocytic leukemia)	$= 0.243 + 0.000403(EN11) + 0.00870(PVH\ Sc) + 0.00536(PH\ Li)$	44.4
TM62F (Acute leukemia)	$= 2.209 - 0.00375(PH\ Mn) - 0.00530(PVH\ Ti) - 0.00881(PH\ F)$	50.7
TM63F (Other leukemia)	$= 0.626 - 0.00256(PL\ B) + 0.00354(PH\ B) - 0.00168(PVH\ Ga)$	53.1
TM64F (All leukemia)	$= 5.129 + 0.213(EN47) + 0.0556(EN48) + 0.00555(PH\ Sr)$	45.8
TM65F (Other and secondary neoplasms)	$= 11.722 - 0.0352(PM\ Mn) - 0.0301(PH\ Sr) - 0.0373(PVL\ As)$	47.6
TM66F (All malignant neoplasms)	$= 119.631 + 0.205(EN5) - 0.108(PVL\ B) - 0.754(PVH\ Nd)$	74.2

See page 49 for key to environmental variables.

or gallium salts is very low. Yet [72]Ga has been proved to concentrate in bone tissues and ^{67}Ga seems to have a tumour-specific affinity.[14]

Non-white Females

Without exception, the stepwise regression equations were able to account for over 50 percent of the variance in the spatial distribution of cancer in non-white females (Table 4,3). The average variance explained was 74.3 percent, while in 21 cases over 80 percent was accounted for. Naturally, the same limitations imposed on the analysis of non-white male mortality by the uneven population distribution of such individuals also applied to non-white females.

Eight environmental variables were found to occur more than three times in the stepwise regression equations. In particular, hay cultivation which appeared nine times and cotton farming which was represented eight times were the most prominent. As noted earlier, this author suspects herbicide use as the possible causal link with cancer. Low levels of iodine, as represented by goitre in troops during World War I, was also selected six times. Other environmental variables that were chosen to appear in the stepwise regression equations, three or more times, included the population of the state, low selenium concentrations in fodder, the amount of sunlight, pollution levels in rivers, and the proportion of the state that was harvested. It would appear, therefore, that exposure to sunlight, inadequate selenium in diet and carcinogens in river water may all play a role in controlling the distribution of cancer in non-white women. However, agricultural carcinogens seem likely to be of predominant significance amongst the environmental variables.

Very high barium is the key soil element that appears to be associated with cancer mortality in non-white females. This potassium antagonist occurred 16 times in the stepwise regression equations. Very low phosphorus levels also appeared six times, while high sodium occurred on seven occasions. Very low potassium was also represented three times, as were medium levels of soil lead. With the exception of lead, the significance of these bulk elements and of barium have already been discussed in detail.

Lead compounds produce mostly renal neoplasms in animals.[15] In humans, chronic lead poisoning tends to affect the central nervous system and the hematopoietic system, as well as the kidney.[16] It should be noted that, as early as 1972, Berg and Burbank suggested that the levels of lead in the drinking water supplies of the United States closely correlated with deaths from lymphomas, all leukemias and renal cancer, regardless of race or sex. In contrast, they argued that mortality from nervous system tumours seemed related to lead only in non-white females.[17]

Table 4,3 Stepwise Multiple Regression Equations — Non-White Females

Dependent Variable	Three Most Significant Independent Variables (0.05 probability level)	Percentage of Total Sum of Squares of Dependent Variable Explained
TM1NWF (Lip)	$= 0.000495 - 0.000646(\text{EN6}) + 0.00254(\text{EN17}) + 0.000895(\text{PH Pb})$	71.3
TM2NWF (Tongue)	$= 0.681 + 0.00151(\text{EN5}) - 0.00852(\text{PVH Ba}) - 0.00400(\text{PVL Mo})$	82.3
TM3NWF (Salivary gland)	$= 0.175 + 0.00338(\text{PM Nb}) - 0.00287(\text{PL Sc}) - 0.00220(\text{PVH As})$	63.9
TM4NWF (Floor of mouth)	$= 0.192 - 0.00477(\text{EN18}) - 0.00134(\text{PVH Al}) - 0.00326(\text{PH Se})$	60.1
TM5NWF (Other mouth)	$= 0.0414 + 0.0211(\text{EN48}) + 0.00678(\text{PL V}) + 0.00576(\text{PVL F})$	72.3
TM6NWF (Oral mesopharynx)	$= -0.109 + 0.00606(\text{EN16}) - 0.00180(\text{PM Co}) + 0.00234(\text{PH Na})$	79.7
TM7NWF (Nasopharynx)	$= -0.311 + 0.000939(\text{EN15}) + 0.0214(\text{EN48}) - 0.0504(\text{EN53})$	76.0
TM8NWF (Hypopharynx)	$= 0.0123 + 0.000147(\text{EN11}) + 0.000569(\text{PL Na}) - 0.00119(\text{PM F})$	54.0
TM9NWF (Pharynx)	$= 0.312 - 0.0193(\text{EN18}) - 0.00297(\text{PH Na}) + 0.00416(\text{PL Li})$	70.0

Table 4.3 (continued)

Dependent Variable	Three Most Significant Independent Variables (0.05 probability level)	Percentage of Total Sum of Squares of Dependent Variable Explained
TM10NWF (Buccal cavity and pharynx)	$= 2.156 - 0.0496(\text{PVH Ba}) - 0.00722(\text{PM Mn}) - 0.0154(\text{PL P})$	76.4
TM11NWF (Esophagus)	$= 2.540 - 0.0156(\text{EN7}) + 0.0318(\text{PH Co}) - 0.0257(\text{PL Hg})$	67.9
TM12NWF (Stomach)	$= 9.696 + 0.0292(\text{PVH Be}) - 0.0403(\text{PM Ce}) + 0.0674(\text{PH Fe})$	58.0
TM13NWF (Small intestine)	$= 0.0578 + 0.0544(\text{EN48}) + 0.00625(\text{PVL Pb}) - 0.00689(\text{PVH Se})$	81.7
TM14NWF (Large intestine)	$= 16.650 - 0.168(\text{EN47}) - 0.224(\text{PVH Ba}) - 0.102(\text{PVL P})$	89.6
TM15NWF (Rectum)	$= 2.564 + 0.00671(\text{EN42}) + 0.0184(\text{EN63}) + 0.0372(\text{PM Mg})$	82.0
TM16NWF (Liver)	$= 8.777 - 0.0167(\text{EN15}) + 0.415(\text{PVH Ba}) - 0.978(\text{PVH Sc})$	90.4
TM17NWF (Pancreas)	$= 7.796 - 0.0752(\text{EN47}) - 0.0197(\text{PM Be}) - 0.0274(\text{PVL K})$	86.5
TM18NWF (Peritoneum)	$= -0.0344 + 0.00331(\text{EN25}) + 0.00274(\text{PH Zr}) + 0.00664(\text{PM Se})$	75.2

Table 4.3 (continued)

Dependent Variable	Three Most Significant Independent Variables (0.05 probability level)	Percentage of Total Sum of Squares of Dependent Variable Explained
TM19NWF (Digestive, unspecified)	$= 0.497 + 0.0236(\text{PVH Ba}) + 0.0130(\text{PL Sc}) + 0.00773(\text{PVL Se})$	56.8
TM20NWF (All digestive)	$= 51.127 - 2.688(\text{EN10}) + 0.0709(\text{PVL Cu}) - 0.296(\text{PVL P})$	90.0
TM21NWF (Nose, middle ear, sinuses)	$= 0.162 - 0.00236(\text{EN12}) + 0.0150(\text{EN18}) + 0.00312(\text{PH As})$	59.8
TM22NWF (Larynx)	$= 0.657 - 0.00429(\text{EN25}) + 0.162(\text{EN53}) - 0.00781(\text{PH Se})$	72.6
TM23NWF (Bronchus, trachea, lung)	$= 1.763 + 0.0000745(\text{EN3}) + 0.105(\text{EN18}) - 0.0230(\text{PL P})$	81.5
TM24NWF (Lung, unspecified)	$= 4.887 - 0.0262(\text{PM Ba}) + 0.0539(\text{PL Mn}) - 0.0430(\text{PVL P})$	74.0
TM25NWF (Mediastinum)	$= 0.0792 - 0.00340(\text{EN12}) + 0.00451(\text{PH Cu}) - 0.00507(\text{PVH Sr})$	60.5
TM26NWF (All respiratory)	$= 7.768 - 0.0738(\text{EN47}) + 0.142(\text{PVH Ba}) - 0.0433(\text{PVL P})$	87.7
TM27NWF (Breast)	$= 25.859 - 0.216(\text{EN47}) - 0.286(\text{PVH B}) - 0.0615(\text{PVL K})$	86.6

Table 4,3 (continued)

Dependent Variable	Three Most Significant Independent Variables (0.05 probability level)	Percentage of Total Sum of Squares of Dependent Variable Explained
TM28NWF (Uterine cervix)	$= 12.826 + 0.755(EN18) + 0.0716(PVL\ Na) + 0.0565(PH\ Ti)$	80.1
TM29NWF (Body of uterus)	$= 0.0990 + 0.0000561(EN3) + 0.210(EN48) + 0.0140(PVL\ Al)$	89.1
TM30NWF (Other uterus)	$= 0.148 + 0.00220(EN35) + 0.00975(EN48) - 0.00235(PVH\ F)$	83.4
TM31NWF (Uterus, unspecified)	$= 10.959 - 0.0248(EN5) - 0.229(PVH\ K) + 0.146(PL\ F)$	71.7
TM32NWF (Ovary)	$= 7.209 - 0.0893(EN47) + 0.0169(PL\ Al) - 0.0200(PVL\ K)$	81.7
TM33NWF (Other female genitals)	$= 1.127 + 0.000666(EN11) - 0.00390(PL\ Sr) - 0.00449(PM\ Yb)$	64.9
TM34NWF (All female genitals)	$= 31.372 + 0.633(EN18) + 0.277(EN28) + 0.0790(PVL\ Na)$	76.3
TM39NWF (Kidney)	$= 1.493 + 0.0275(EN35) + 0.0127(PM\ Pb) - 0.0106(PVL\ Sr)$	74.9
TM40NWF (Bladder)	$= 3.002 + 0.00747(EN5) + 0.0324(PVH\ Mo) - 0.0351(PM\ Ti)$	70.0

Table 4.3 (continued)

Dependent Variable	Three Most Significant Independent Variables (0.05 probability level)	Percentage of Total Sum of Squares of Dependent Variable Explained
TM41NWF (All urinary tract)	= 5.480 − 0.0335(PVL Mn) + 0.0271(PVL Yb) − 0.0346(PL Hg)	75.0
TM42NWF (Melanoma)	= 0.322 − 0.0105(PVH Ba) + 0.00400(PH Na) − 0.00316(PM Y)	68.7
TM43NWF (Skin)	= 0.695 − 0.0143(PVH Ba) − 0.00711(PM Co) + 0.00361(PM Nd)	67.0
TM44NWF (Entire Integument)	= 0.765 + 0.00970(EN17) − 0.0306(PVH Ba) + 0.00607(PH Na)	72.0
TM45NWF (Eye)	= −0.308 + 3.343(EN29) + 0.0132(PL Pb) + 0.00222(PVH Pb)	78.2
TM46NWF (Nervous system)	= 2.0665 − 0.0554(PVH Ba) − 0.00675(PM Sc) − 0.00796(PVL Na)	81.6
TM47NWF (Thyroid)	= 2.497 − 0.00446(EN15) + 0.0659(PVH Ba) − 0.00603(PM Pb)	89.7
TM48NWF (Bone)	= 1.057 − 0.00539(PH Ba) − 0.0174(PVH Ba) − 0.00803(PH Na)	74.5
TM49NWF (Connective Tissue)	= 0.279 + 0.0196(EN28) − 0.0118(PH Co) + 0.00472(PM Se)	59.8

111

Table 4.3 (continued)

Dependent Variable	Three Most Significant Independent Variables (0.05 probability level)	Percentage of Total Sum of Squares of Dependent Variable Explained
TM50NWF (Reticulum cell sarcoma)	$= 0.0467 + 0.000483(\text{EN42}) + 0.0308(\text{EN48}) + 0.00226(\text{PVL B})$	74.0
TM51NWF (Lymphosarcoma)	$= 0.611 - 0.0166(\text{EN47}) + 0.0101(\text{PL Al}) + 0.00544(\text{PM Ni})$	68.9
TM52NWF (Other lymphoid neoplasms)	$= 0.383 + 0.0217(\text{PVH Ba}) - 0.00322(\text{PH Na}) - 0.00222(\text{PVL Sr})$	78.9
TM53NWF (Hodgkin's disease)	$= 0.604 + 0.0365(\text{EN48}) - 0.00347(\text{PM Nd}) + 0.00829(\text{PM Sr})$	83.7
TM54NWF (Giant follicular lymphoma)	$= 0.0888 - 0.000480(\text{PVL Pb}) - 0.000823(\text{PVL Mo}) + 0.000337(\text{PVL Sr})$	63.7
TM55NWF (Other reticuloses)	$= 0.639 - 0.00633(\text{EN8}) - 0.0154(\text{PVH Ba}) - 0.00320(\text{PH Ni})$	65.5
TM56NWF (Mycosis fungoides)	$= 0.0566 - 0.00328(\text{PVH Ba}) + 0.00212(\text{PH Na}) - 0.000592(\text{PM Yb})$	71.4
TM57NWF (Multiple myeloma)	$= 2.633 - 0.00558(\text{EN25}) - 0.0454(\text{EN47}) - 0.00937(\text{PVL Mg})$	82.1
TM58NWF (All lymphomas)	$= 5.753 - 0.0675(\text{EN47}) - 0.0144(\text{PH Pb}) - 0.0296(\text{PVL P})$	90.6

Table 4.3 (continued)

Dependent Variable	Three Most Significant Independent Variables (0.05 probability level)	Percentage of Total Sum of Squares of Dependent Variable Explained
TM59NWF (Lymphatic leukemia)	$= 0.791 + 0.0000246(EN3) - 0.0328(PVH\ Ba) - 0.00516(PL\ Yb)$	63.2
TM60NWF (Myeloid leukemia)	$= 1.089 - 0.232(EN19) + 0.0736(EN48) - 0.00592(PM\ Pb)$	83.2
TM61NWF (Monocytic leukemia)	$= 0.475 - 0.00247(EN21) + 0.0243(EN40) - 0.0202(PVH\ Ba)$	61.1
TM62NWF (Acute leukemia)	$= 0.680 + 0.0000279(EN3) + 0.00654(EN63) + 0.00417(PM\ Ca)$	71.2
TM63NWF (Other leukemia)	$= 0.608 + 0.00468(EN54A) + 0.00354(PM\ B) - 0.0101(PL\ Fe)$	64.5
TM64NWF (All leukemia)	$= 3.973 - 0.844(EN19) + 0.00466(EN22) + 0.154(EN48)$	73.5
TM65NWF (Other and secondary neoplasms)	$= 20.066 - 0.196(EN28) - 0.0854(PVL\ Cu) - 0.0918(PVH\ Ga)$	64.4
TM66NWF (All malignant neoplasms)	$= 168.303 - 6.134(EN10) - 0.508(PVL\ P) - 0.200(PM\ Zn)$	84.1

See page 49 for key to environmental variables.

113

CONCLUSIONS

The stepwise regression equations tend to confirm the tentative previous conclusions reached as a result of the use of Pearson correlation coefficients. They also suggest that cancer mortality in the United States reflects the distribution of industrial and agricultural carcinogens, together with the positive and negative impacts of certain naturally occurring soil elements. In particular, stepwise regression highlights the significance of the bulk and trace elements calcium, sodium, potassium, manganese, zinc, iodine and selenium, together with the antagonists barium and strontium. Barium seems especially important as a carcinogen in non-whites. Also of interest is the repeated appearance in the stepwise regression equations, for certain sexes or races, of the suspected carcinogens, arsenic, chromium, mercury and lead. The author is less able to explain the roles of gallium, fluorine, boron and lanthanum, but the associations between these elements and cancer appear to warrant further exploration. Of course, their appearance in these equations may simply reflect the operation of chance.

REFERENCES

1. JOHNSTON, R.J., *Multivariate Statistical Analysis in Geography: A Primer on the General Linear Model*. London: Longmans, 1980, pp. 84-87.

2. TIDBALL, R.R. and SAVER, H.I., "Multivariate Relationships Between Soil Composition and Human Mortality Rates in Missouri". In FREEDMAN, J. (ed.), *Trace Element Geochemistry in Health and Disease*. The Geological Society of America Special Paper 155, 1975, pp. 41-59.

3. MARK, D.M. and PEUCKER, T.K., "Regression Analysis and Geographic Models". *Canadian Geographer*, vol. XXIII(1), 1979, pp. 51-64.

4. TIDBALL and SAVER, *op. cit.*, pp. 51-55.

5. SNEDECOR, G.W. and COCHRAN, W.G., *Statistical Methods*, 6th Edition. Ames: Iowa State University Press, 1967, 593 pp.

6. TIDBALL and SAVER, *op. cit.*, pp. 51-55.

7. BERG, J.W. and BURBANK, F., "Correlations Between Carcinogenic Trace Metals in Water Supplies and Cancer Mortality". *Annals, New York Academy of Sciences*, vol. 199, 1972, pp. 249-265.

8. SPEDDING, F.H., "Rare Earth Elements". *Encyclopedia of Chemical Technology*, vol. 19. New York: John Wiley, 1982, pp. 833-838.

9. *Ibid.*, pp. 850-851.

10. *Ibid.*

11. BERG and BURBANK, *op. cit.*, p. 249.

12. LINDAHL, C.B. and MESHRI, D.T., "Fluorine Compounds — Inorganic". *Encyclopedia of Chemical Technology*, vol. 10. New York: John Wiley, 1980, p. 658.

13. DOONAN, D.J. and LOWER, L.D., "Boron Compounds (Oxides, Acid, Borates)". *Encyclopedia of Chemical Technology*, vol. 4. New York: John Wiley, 1978, p. 96.

14. DE LA BRETÈQUE, P., "Gallium and Gallium Compounds". *Encyclopedia of Chemical Technology*, vol. 11. New York: John Wiley, 1980, pp. 618-619.

15. BOYLAND, E., DUKES, C.E., GROVER, P.L. and MITCHLEY, C.V., "The Induction of Renal Tumours by Feeding Lead Acetate to Rats". *British Journal of Cancer*, vol. 16, 1962, pp. 283-288.

16. GOYER, R.A., "Lead Toxicity: A Problem in Environmental Pathology". *American Journal of Pathology*, vol. 64, 1971, pp. 167-180.

17. BERG and BURBANK, *op. cit.*, p. 255.

*Cancer is a complex of diseases induced
primarily by the action of environmental
agents on susceptible hosts. Currently, the
only way known to prevent human cancers
is by preventing or minimizing exposures to
these environmental agents.*

Robert Hoover, 1979

*It is estimated that 53 million people now
alive in the country [U.S.A.] will eventually
have cancer, and 35 million people will die
from it, unless new methods of prevention,
treatment or cures are found.*

National Health Education Committee, 1976

4 GLOBAL OVERVIEW

TESTING THE HYPOTHESES

The scientific method involves more than analysis, hypothesis genera-
tion and prediction. It must also include checking theory against reality,
so that its validity can be assessed and any necessary modifications made.
Biochemists undertake this process in the laboratory, while the medical
profession tests its ideas in hospital wards. Geographers, in contrast, must
use variations in spatial patterns as a proving ground for their hypotheses.
For this reason, the author now examines the global distribution of several
major specific cancers, with a view to testing the validity, or otherwise, of
the hypotheses generated by the statistical analysis of United States cancer
mortality data. Obviously, in a publication of this nature, not all specific
cancers can be assessed in this manner. Attention, therefore, has been
limited to six, namely those of the liver, esophagus, stomach, breast,
uterine cervix, and melanoma. At least five of these, when viewed globally
are amongst the most deadly.[1]

Cancer of the Liver, Esophagus and Stomach

The statistical analysis of mortality data from the United States suggests
that cancer of the esophagus is associated with a diet containing too little
selenium and calcium and too much sodium (Table 2,2). If this hypothesis
is correct, esophageal cancer is most likely to be prevalent, on a global
scale, in those countries, or regions, where the water is very soft, that is,
where it contains little calcium. Esophageal cancer will also be common
where salt is very prevalent, because of the presence of salt domes, or
high evaporation rates (which concentrate sodium chloride in upper soil
horizons), or because of the excessive use of salt in cooking, or of highway
de-icing compounds. Conversely, if cancer of the liver is associated with
the damage caused by long term exposure to too much calcium and
magnesium, it will tend to peak in hard water regions, especially if calcium
and magnesium enriched foods form a significant part of diet

It follows, therefore, that the spatial distributions of cancer of the esophagus and of the liver ought to be inversely related, high mortality rates from
both rarely being found in the same region. One should not expect this

relationship to be absolute, since potassium also appears to play a significant role in mortality from cancer of the liver. Exceptions may occur in regions where beer is consumed to excess, because this will elevate serum potassium levels, probably giving rise to liver cancer, even in soft water areas (Table 2,2). One would expect, therefore, that the inverse relationship between esophageal and liver cancers would be most obvious in women, who consume less beer than their male counterparts.

In contrast, since cancer of the stomach appears related to high dietary intake of potassium and sodium, mortality from this specific cancer ought to have a fairly similar distribution to that of the esophagus. This is because calcium deficient areas are also likely to be enriched in sodium and potassium. Potassium occurs in the feldspars and micas of igneous rocks, while its compounds are common in evaporites.[2] There are also commercial potassium operations on the Dead Sea and Great Salt Lake. In many of those deposits potassium is closely associated with sodium chloride.[3] Conversely, calcium is likely to be very deficient in both potassium rich igneous rocks and in sodium and potassium enriched evaporites. Calcium does not appear with sodium and potassium in evaporites because of differences in solubility, calcium being precipitated earlier than sodium in the sequence.

Fortunately the global distribution of esophageal,[4] stomach[5] and liver[6] cancers have recently been reviewed. The world's highest incidence and/or mortality rates for esophageal cancer, on a national level, appear to occur amongst Bulawayo African males in Zimbabwe and Natal African males in South Africa, where rates are 63.8 and 40.9, per year, per 100,000. The lowest levels are found in countries such as Nigeria and Romania, where they reach only 1.5 and 1.9, per year, per 100,000 amongst males.[7] Age standardized death rates per 100,000 from cancer of the stomach are highest amongst males in Japan, 54.5 per 100,000 annually; and lowest in Thailand and Nicaragua where they are 1.4 and 1.9 per 100,000, per year, in males.[8] Senegal also has very low age standardized incidence rates for stomach cancer, 3.7 for men and 2.0 for women.

While Cook-Mozaffari and van Rensburg[9] do not discuss liver cancer mortality for all of these countries, it is described for South African white males. In contrast to their exceedingly high mortality from esophageal cancer, these individuals have amongst the world's lowest age standardized incidence levels for primary liver cancer, less than 4 per 100,000. South African coloreds and Indians also have a very low level of incidence of this disease, between 4 and 12 per 100,000 annually. Northern Japan has a slightly higher incidence of primary liver cancer, between 12 and 25 per 100,000 per year. Nigeria and Senegal have elevated liver cancer rates as does Zimbabwe.[10]

With the exception of Zimbabwe, the predicted inverse relationship between cancers of the esophagus and stomach and of the liver appear to hold true on a global scale. The situation in Zimbabwe seems to reflect excessive beer consumption and, therefore, very elevated potassium levels. To quote Schapera and Goodwin,[11]

> Beer is regarded by the Bantu as an essential food. In times of plenty it is not only freely consumed, but often is the principal or even sole food for many men for days on end. But it also plays a very important part in their social life. The whole social system of the people is inextricably linked up with this popular beverage, which is the first essential of all festivities, the one incentive to labor, the first thought in dispensing hospitality, the favorite tribute of subjects to their chief, and almost the only votive offering dedicated to their spirits.

At the regional level, the publication of various atlases of mortality permit cancers of the esophagus, stomach and liver to be compared. As can be seen from Figure 1,4, in the People's Republic of China, male cancers of the esophagus and stomach show fairly similar distribution patterns, while that of liver cancer is extremely different (Figures 2,4 and 3,4), there being very little overlap between high levels of liver cancer and elevated levels of cancer of the esophagus and of the stomach.[12] This relationship was tested statistically using data available in the atlas, establishing a negative correlation between cancer of the esophagus and liver (r = −0.47054, p = 0.01); and stomach and liver (r = −0.50402, p = 0.0053) in Chinese males. Considering the very large regions involved these negative correlations are seen as supportive of the hypotheses.

British cancer distributions have been illustrated in the *Atlas of Cancer Mortality in England and Wales, 1968-1978*[13] and discussed in some detail by Gardner.[14] Unfortunately, while the maps of mortality from cancer of the esophagus and stomach are produced for each local authority, that of the liver is illustrated at the county level. This difference in mapping scale makes comparison difficult. However, there appears to be quite strong confirming evidence for the postulated reversed relationship between cancers of the esophagus and liver. For example, in women, mortality from cancer of the esophagus is particularly high in Wales and Cornwall. In liver cancer, the reverse appears true (Figure 4,4). The situation appears more confused in males, again perhaps because of high beer, and hence potassium, consumption.

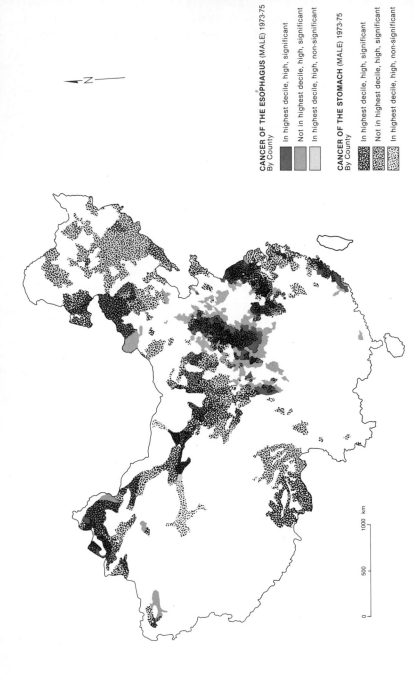

CANCER OF THE ESOPHAGUS (MALE) 1973-75
By County

In highest decile, high, significant

Not in highest decile, high, significant

In highest decile, high, non-significant

CANCER OF THE STOMACH (MALE) 1973-75
By County

In highest decile, high, significant

Not in highest decile, high, significant

In highest decile, high, non-significant

Figure 1.4 A Comparison of Mortality from Cancer of the Stomach and Esophagus in Males, in the People's Republic of China (1973-1975)

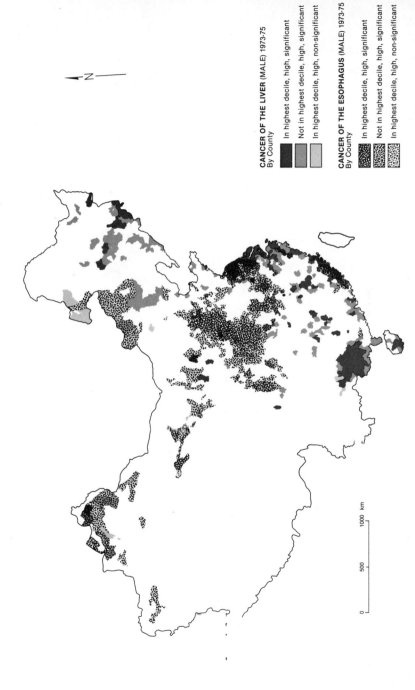

CANCER OF THE LIVER (MALE) 1973-75
By County

In highest decile, high, significant

Not in highest decile, high, significant

In highest decile, high, non-significant

CANCER OF THE ESOPHAGUS (MALE) 1973-75
By County

In highest decile, high, significant

Not in highest decile, high, significant

In highest decile, high, non-significant

N

0   500   1000 km

Figure 2.4 A Comparison of Mortality from Cancer of the Esophagus and Liver in Males, in the People's Republic of China (1973-1975)

123

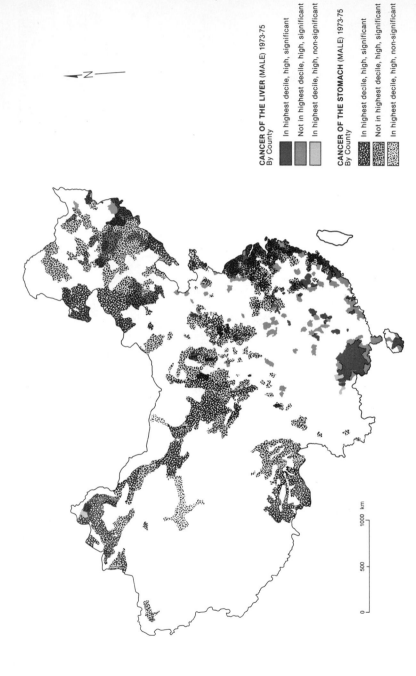

CANCER OF THE LIVER (MALE) 1973-75
By County

In highest decile, high, significant

Not in highest decile, high, significant

In highest decile, high, non-significant

CANCER OF THE STOMACH (MALE) 1973-75
By County

In highest decile, high, significant

Not in highest decile, high, significant

In highest decile, high, non-significant

Figure 3.4 A Comparison of Mortality from Cancer of the Stomach and Liver in Males, in the People's Republic of China (1973-1975)

124

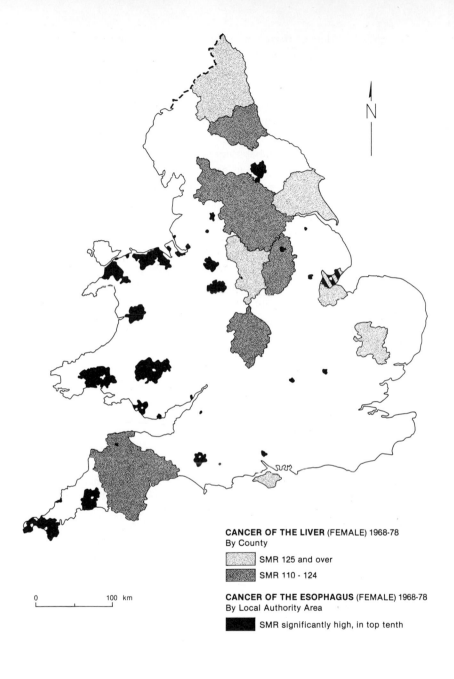

CANCER OF THE LIVER (FEMALE) 1968-78
By County

SMR 125 and over

SMR 110 - 124

CANCER OF THE ESOPHAGUS (FEMALE) 1968-78
By Local Authority Area

SMR significantly high, in top tenth

0   100 km

Figure 4,4   A Comparison of Mortality from Cancer of the Esophagus and Liver
in Females, in England and Wales (1968-1978)

125

The global evidence, therefore, would seem to confirm the hypothesis that high calcium levels tend to prevent cancer of the esophagus, while simultaneously encouraging development of liver cancer. Blurring of this relationship appears to occur because of excessive beer consumption amongst some males, which results in very elevated potassium levels, which in themselves apparently encourage mortality from cancer of the liver and stomach.

There is also extensive global evidence that cancers of the esophagus and stomach are very common in areas where water is soft and saline. In England and Wales, for example, if a line is drawn from Redcar (which lies to the south of Middlesbrough in Durham) to the mouth of the River Severn, it divides England and Wales roughly into half. That region to the west might be termed the highlands and that to the east the lowlands. It can be seen from Gardner's[15] map of male cancer of the stomach that some 90 percent of all local authority areas with standardized mortality ratios that are significantly low, and in the bottom decile, are located to the east of this line in the lowlands. In contrast, some 80 percent of those authority areas with standardized mortality ratios that are significantly high and in the top decile, lie to the west, in the highlands (Figures 5,4 and 6,4).

This author has subjected this distribution of male stomach cancer to point pattern analysis, using a grid containing 27 cells.[16] Variance/mean ratios of 4.400 and 3.152 were obtained for the distribution of local authorities that had significantly high (in the top tenth) and significantly low (in the bottom tenth) standardized mortality ratios for male stomach cancer during the period 1968 to 1978. These variance/mean ratios clearly show that the distributions of high and low levels of mortality from stomach cancer in Britain are very clustered. Using the Student's t-test for statistical significance it was established that the possibility that the distribution is random can be rejected with a probability > 0.001. Clearly, both clustered distributions are highly significant. It is of interest to note that, in Britain, male cancer of the buccal cavity also shows a very similar mortality pattern.[17] The only major exception to this generalization occurs in an administrative region called Parts of Holland, in Lincolnshire, which includes the Spalding area. This is one of the few regions in Eastern England (Humberside, Lincolnshire, Norfolk and Suffolk) that is not closely associated with the Chalk, the latter having been eroded by the Wash. The bulk of the population, therefore, lives on the Oxford Clay.[18]

Indeed it is apparent that differences in the occurrence of male stomach and buccal cavity cancer mortality in England and Wales are not merely geographical. They also clearly reflect geological influence. For example, when the male stomach cancer maps of England and Wales, produced by

Gardner *et al.*,[19] are placed side by side with those in the Wolfson Geochemical Atlas[20] which illustrate the spatial distribution of potassium and calcium in some 50,000 stream bed sediments, an immediate visual correlation is obvious. With a few minor exceptions, the Redcar-Severn line divides the calcium enriched potassium deficient east from the calcium deficient potassium enriched west. Similarly, when the male, and indeed the female, stomach cancer mortality maps are compared with the *Ordnance Survey "Ten Mile" Geological Maps of Great Britain*, correlations are immediately apparent.[21] Significantly low mortality from cancer of the stomach is found almost exclusively in counties located on, or receiving drainage from such calcium rich rocks as the Permian Magnesium limestone, the Carboniferous limestone and the Cretaceous chalk. For example, significantly low levels occur on the chalk of the Yorkshire Wolds, Lincolnshire Wolds, East Anglia, the Chiltern Hills and North and South Downs (Figure 6,4). Concentrations of calcium carbonate, in water draining from such British chalk and limestone areas, commonly fall into the range of 150 to 250 ppm.[22] In contrast, significantly high levels of male stomach cancer mortality are found in local authorities located in the Lleyn Peninsula, Snowdonia, the English Lake District, the Pennines and Tyne and Teeside. These are predominantly soft water areas, deficient in calcium, but rich in potassium, because their rivers rise in areas of shale, slate, grits, rhyolites, breccias and tuffs, all of which are Palaeozoic calcium-deficient rocks. Indeed, the soft water of the Carboniferous Millstone Grits and Coal Measures was a major reason why the textile industry located in the Lancashire and Yorkshire Pennines, at the beginning of the Industrial Revolution.

The author is aware that finished water often differs chemically from that of the streams, reservoirs and aquifers used to supply the delivery system. Treatment plants, for example, may increase or decrease hardness, add fluorine and/or chlorine and remove sodium and suspended sediment before supplying their markets.[23] To illustrate, the Severn-Trent Water Authority sets a maximum total hardness standard of 100 ppm and consistently softens water to reach this level before supplying it to consumers.[24] In contrast, Manchester hardened soft water it was receiving from the Lake District by adding lime.[25] Of course, soft water may also be transported to hard water areas by aqueducts, or vice versa. The development of the Yorkshire Water Grid, for example, was expected to result in water of differing hardness being transferred to areas which traditionally had been supplied with either hard or soft water. In the Hull region, for instance, the use of some water from the grid was expected to result in a marginal reduction in water hardness.[26]

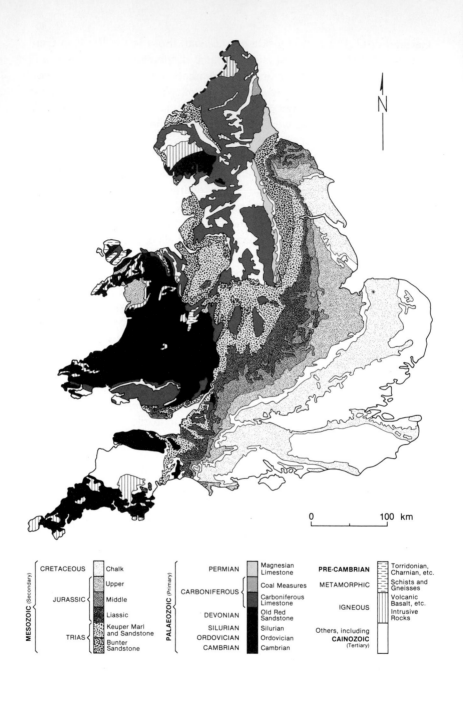

Figure 5,4 A Generalized Geological Map of England and Wales

128

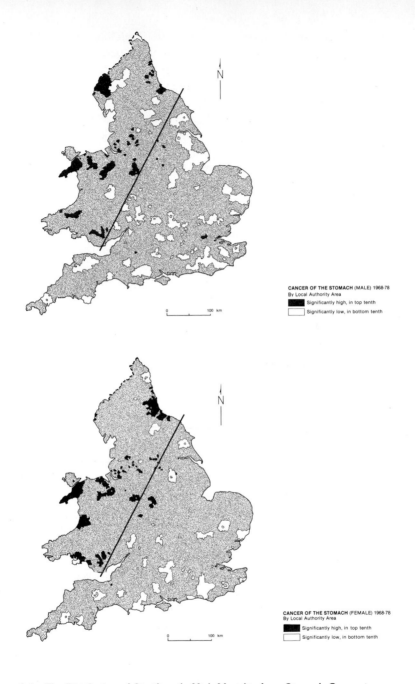

Figure 6,4 The Distribution of Significantly High Mortality from Stomach Cancer in Males and Females in England and Wales (1968-1978)

129

It is dangerous to generalize too much, therefore, about the hardness of water actually drunk on the basis of geological maps alone. However, natural differences in water hardness in Britain are so marked that treatment is unlikely to do more than blur regional characteristics and the geological map and the Wolfson Geochemical Atlas[27] still provide a realistic impression of probable differences in the calcium, potassium and sodium content of domestic water supplies. To check this fact, the author wrote to every major water supply agency in England and Wales, asking for analyses of drinking water quality. Chemical analyses from hundreds of wells, rivers and lakes were supplied. Water to the west of the Redcar-Severn line is generally very soft, while that to the east is normally hard and calcium enriched. For example, in Wales, rivers such as the Rheidol and Ystwyth, that rise on Silurian mudstones and greywackes have very low total hardness, in this case 9 and 19 ppm respectively.[28] Conversely, to the east of the Redcar-Severn dividing line, water taken from aquifers often has a high carbonate hardness; that from the Inferior Oolite, Great Oolite and Chalk in the Thames Conservancy, for instance, averaging some 195, 255, and 215 ppm respectively. By way of contrast, the water from aquifers in the Lower Greensand has an average carbonate hardness of only 84 ppm.[29]

These apparent relationships between low mortality from esophageal cancer and high calcium exposure and high mortality and low calcium intake can also be demonstrated elsewhere in Europe. Here the major patterns of variation are seen for males, the incidence for females being low or very low over most of the continent. Contrasts amongst males are particularly striking in Brittany, Normandy and Italy. These distributions were illustrated by Day, who provided maps showing differences in age standardized mortality rates per 100,000, for cancer of the esophagus among males, for the period 1958 to 1966, for all three regions.[30]

In western and eastern Brittany, most cantons have male mortality rates similar to the rest of France, that is 14 percent per 100,000. In central Brittany, the focus of highest mortality, the rates may be five to ten times higher.[31] Brittany consists primarily of Palaeozoic slates, shales and other calcium deficient rocks, similar to those of North Wales. However, there is also a central spine of Permian and Carboniferous deposits, which cross the peninsula from west to east. Limestones within these sediments are highly calcareous, giving rise, for example, to a calcium rich spring near Saint-Servan, which is significant enough to be shown on the *Carte Des Eaux Minérales et Thermales De La France*.[32] These Carboniferous rocks are not continuous, however, and there is approximately a 160 kilometre gap in central Brittany where they do not occur, or are very restricted. When the geological map of Brittany is compared with that of

130

esophageal cancer mortality, it is very apparent that those cantons receiving calcium enriched drainage that rises on the Carboniferous limestone rocks of western and eastern Brittany have low esophageal cancer mortalities, the abnormally high rates occurring only in cantons in central Brittany where these limestones are absent. Even within this belt of excessive mortality there are more affected cantons in the north than in the south. This distribution appears to reflect the course of the Vilaine, which has its headwaters in the Carboniferous rock of eastern Brittany and then flows southwestwards to enter the Bay of Biscay near La Roche-Bernard.

Male esophageal cancer mortality patterns in the Normandy departments of Calvados and Orne show similar large variations.[33] The highest mortality rates, over 50 per 100,000, occurring in the west, except along the north coast of Normandy where rates are moderate or low. Mortality also drops off sharply in eastern Normandy, reaching levels that are usually between 0 to 19.9 per 100,000. The geology of Normandy is quite complex, the western cantons lying on the same calcium deficient Palaeozoic rocks found throughout most of Brittany. Along the northern coast, however, Jurassic and Cretaceous rocks occur, while in the east, Normandy is dominated by Cretaceous chalks. Deterministic though it may seem, the crenulated boundary between high and low esophageal cancer mortality follows the unconformity between the Palaeozoic and Mesozoic sediments very closely, high mortality cantons occurring farthest east to the south of Lisieux, where the Palaeozoic reaches its maximum eastward penetration into northern Normandy.

It Italy, even though esophageal cancer rates nowhere reach the levels seen in Brittany, there are still marked spatial variations in male mortality. Between the northeast and the south there is a sixfold difference.[34] The highest rates are found on the Palaeozoic rocks of the northeast, while the lowest mortality coincides with the distribution of Mesozoic rocks, levels apparently reaching their lowest in the "heel" of Italy. In this area, between Bari and Brindisi, there is a large outcrop of Cretacious chalk.[35]

The world's most striking geographical distribution of male esophageal cancer is the Central Asian high incidence belt. This consists of parts of northern China and regions of extremely elevated mortality in Kazakhstan, Uzbekistan and Turkmenistan in the Soviet Union. Also included are the northeast of Iran and northern Afghanistan. The author has examined the geology of these areas using maps from three Chinese and Russian sources.[36] It is immediately apparent that in all of these countries, exceptionally high areas of mortality from esophageal cancer coincide with the great Quaternary loess and sand belts of Asia. Such deposits are aeolian, having been deposited by the wind, either on the margins of desert and semi-desert areas, or in periglacial environments beyond major ice sheets.

131

Aeolian sands consist of particles, usually 0.06 to 1.0 millimetres in diameter, that are predominantly composed of quartz grains. Aeolian silt, generally known as loess, is buff colored, well-sorted, with particle sizes between 0.01 and 0.05 millimetres.[37] High levels of esophageal cancer throughout Central Asia appear to correlate very well with the regional distribution of these sediments, especially high mortality occurring in areas dominated by wind-blown Quaternary sands.[38]

There is a very complete water quality monitoring network in the Soviet Union. In 1967, for example, Pavelko and Tarasov[39] produced hydrochemical maps of the rivers of the Kazakhstan. These were based on data from 290 water quality monitoring stations at which samples had been taken for over 25 years. Even so, stations were relatively scarce in many of the areas of high esophageal cancer mortality, because of the great permeability of loess and sand and the high temperatures and evaporation rates which resulted in very restricted surface drainage. Nevertheless, it is clear from the maps produced that, in areas of aeolian deposition and high cancer mortality, the salinity of the water is very high and the ion concentrations (including that of calcium) are low. Pavelko and Tarasov[40] provide numerous graphs, based on thousands of water quality observations, that indicate there is an inverse relationship between water salinity and both bicarbonates and calcium. As the sodium content of water in the Kazakhstan increases, its calcium content declines. Saline waters, therefore, are low in both bicarbonates and calcium. Salinity tends to be highest where evaporation rates are excessive and soils are sandy or silty. Here salt is drawn to the surface through capillary action.[41] This occurs in areas like the Kazakhstan which have low rates of precipitation and, therefore, where the soils are not heavily leached. Pavelko and Tarasov[42] demonstrate that throughout this area, the calcium content of river water rarely exceeds 40 ppm and is generally less than 20 ppm. In contrast, maximum annual mineralization of some of the rivers of Kazakhstan reaches as high as 78,000 ppm, mainly because of the high sodium and chloride content. Inhabitants of the Kazakhstan, because of geology and climate, must almost inevitably drink water that is calcium deficient and very saline. This may also explain the patterns of esophageal cancer in the Caspian littoral of Iran, described by Kmet and Mahboubi.[43] Rainfall in the east of this area is only one-quarter of that in the west. As might be expected, the highest mortality from esophageal cancer is associated with the resultant saline soils which are found in the east.

Over 60 percent of the global incidence of esophageal cancer occurs in the People's Republic of China.[44] Here it is the second most common cancer, behind that of the stomach (Figure 1,4). The national annual mortality rate for these two cancers is very similar, 32.5 per 100,000 in males and 15.9 in females for stomach cancer, and 31.7 for men and 15.9 for women from cancer of the esophagus.[45] The distribution of these diseases differs somewhat, although extremes tend to be located in the same areas. Stomach cancer is more common in the north than the south. So too is esophageal cancer (Figure 1,4). However, changes in incidence are relatively smooth for stomach cancer. Esophageal cancer, in contrast, is rare over large tracts of the country, the disease being found in a few sharply demarcated areas, in which mortality levels are considerably higher than seen anywhere for cancer of the stomach.[46] To summarize, levels of both stomach and esophageal cancer are lowest in the Great Plain of China, the mountains of South China and the Xijiang Valley. Since these areas include many of the People's Republic of China's largest cities and industrial complexes, for example Beijing, Tianjin and Guangzhou, it cannot be argued that there is any very strong correlation between high stomach and esophageal cancer mortality rates and man-made pollution.[47]

The distribution of stomach and esophageal cancer appears to show a far closer visual correlation with the geology and hydrology of that country than with its industrial base. High mortality rates such as those in Qigihar, adjoining Mongolia and Hingan, abutting the Soviet Union, tend to occur in areas of Holocene aeolian sands and Pleistocene loess.[48] Mortalities appear particularly high in such areas where the underlying bedrock is of potassium-rich calcium-poor igneous origin, for example basalts, granites, andesites or trachytes. In contrast, lower incidence rates, particularly for esophageal cancer, are clustered in areas of Ordovician, Triassic, Jurassic and Cretacious limestones, as, for example, on the Shandong peninsula. Low mortality in southern China also appears to reflect the presence of large areas of Triassic and Permian limestone in the western tributaries of the Xijiang, while Devonian limestone also outcrops further east. In addition, Archean marbles tend to be prevalent in many regions of low mortality, as, for example, in the eastern section of the Huanghe Valley.[49] The low mortality rates for both stomach and esophageal cancer in the western ranges of the mountains of South China, in Guizhou, appear to coincide with extensive outcrops of Triassic limestones and shales.

These differences in geology are, of course, reflected in the water quality of the People's Republic of China. Knowledge of this is relatively limited, although Hsieh[50] has published two summary maps in the *Atlas of China*, illustrating water hardness and chloride and bicarbonate content. It would appear that high esophageal cancer mortality is most common in the People's Republic of China in areas where the water is both relatively soft and highly saline. In addition, it is thought that excessive salt is also used in food preparation in many of these areas.

Although the People's Republic of China has the largest absolute number of esophageal cancer deaths, incidence and mortality rates both peak amongst the Bantu males of Zimbabwe where, interestingly enough, female rates are very low. Day[51] gives incidence and mortality rates per year per 100,000 as 63.8 for males and 2.2 for females in this country.

Zimbabwe has a radial drainage system, because of its mountainous core, and water consumed within its borders is almost invariably from internal sources. Since the geology of Zimbabwe consists almost entirely of Archaean greenstones and ironstones, granites, paragneisses, basaltic lavas, sandstones and shales, there is virtually no source of calcium.[52]

The Bantu typically keep herds of cattle and goats. However, in the higher parts of southern Africa such as Zimbabwe, grazing may be relatively poor and milk yields reduced. Under these circumstances, the milk products are primarily eaten by women and children. Menstruating women, however, are not permitted to eat milk products by taboo. This, of course, ensures that pregnant wives receive a larger share. There are many other food taboos that influence diet.[53] Beer is also regarded by the Bantu as an essential food. They brew a wide range of such intoxicating liquors, usually reserving the strongest for males.[54]

From this brief description of the geography of Zimbabwe, the causes of the world's highest esophageal cancer rates may perhaps be surmised. The bedrock of Zimbabwe is calcium deficient and its topography and radial drainage ensures that this element is not "imported" from outside sources. Bantu customs and food taboos have traditionally promoted the consumption of relatively calcium rich, milk dominated diets by women and children, and calcium poor, beer dominated diets by males.

In contrast, the world's lowest age standardized mortality and incidence rates for cancer of the esophagus appear to occur in Romania, where Day[55] reports 1.9 and 0.5 per year per 100,000, for males and females respectively. Romania's geology is very calcareous with chalk forming a major component of the bedrock of the Carpathian Mountains. Other calcareous rocks such as limestone and dolomite are common. As a result, the production of cement, quicklime and plaster is spread throughout Romania, the country's largest cement mill being located at Tîrgu Jiu. Marble is also quarried at Ruschita and Caprioara, Alun and Văscău.[56]

Romania has been perhaps Europe's major centre for health resorts and spas since Roman times.[57] There are some 2,000 mineral springs in the country and the health spas of Romania are under the direct supervision of the Institute of Balneology and Physiotherapy, which has made a detailed study of their therapeutic qualities. The water at Herculane in the Cerna Valley, for example, is noted for its bicarbonates, calcium, sulphur and sodium chloride. It is considered that this spa is suitable for the treatment of rheumatism and diseases of the gastro-intestinal tract and liver. Eforie Nord, situated on the Black Sea coast, is promoted as a centre for the treatment of rickets, among other ailments.[58] The Romanians drink enormous quantities of calcium enriched mineral water since, as Latham[59] points out, "the water in Romania is drinkable with safety, though there is rarely any need to drink it because mineral waters are provided everywhere free of charge with all meals, even breakfast".

In contrast, the world's highest age standardized incidence and mortality rates for stomach cancer are recorded in Japan.[60] Incidence in Miyagi, for example, reaches 88.0 per 100,000 per year in men and 42.0 annually for women. The islands of Japan are the projecting summits of a major mountain chain which was originally part of the Asian continent. Topographically, Japan is a rugged land of high mountains, which include some 200 volcanoes dissected by deep valleys. Soils are rocky and only an estimated 15 to 18 percent of Japan is arable. No part of Japan is more than 160 kilometres from the sea. Most of the rocks are volcanic or igneous. As a consequence, river water in Japan is relatively soft and low in calcium, the average hardness being less than 40 ppm, compared with the United States where the mean hardness of raw municipal water is 139 ppm.[61] In an effort to discover information on the potassium content of drinking water in Japan the author conducted a computer search of Selected Water Resource Abstracts. One hundred and fifty-two titles were retrieved and numerous abstracts reviewed. Nevertheless, the information available is incomplete. Calcium levels are clearly very low, but there is little published information on potassium in drinking water. While the author has been unable to find adequate water quality data, it seems reasonable to assume on the basis of geology that potassium levels are high.

Because of their proximity to the sea, extended shoreline, large population and relatively small potential for agriculture, the Japanese eat large quantities of fish. It is a staple food, second only in importance to rice. Livestock is relatively unimportant to Japanese agriculture, because arable land is scarce and valuable, so that little can be devoted to dairying.

The soft water in Japan is a poor source of calcium; so, too, is rice when grown in volcanic soils. Since dairying is rare, little milk, cheese or yogurt is consumed. Fish is also a poor source of calcium, except when eaten whole, as in the case of sardines.[62] The Japanese diet, therefore, is generally very low in calcium.

In contrast, however, the Japanese consume very large quantities of salt (⩾15 g NaCl/day), a level which is amongst the world's highest.[53] A major reason for this is their widespread use of soy sauce, the primary seasoning of Japanese cooking, which is made from soy beans and salt.[64]

135

Interestingly, Joossens and Geboers[65] observed a strong correlation between stroke and gastric cancer mortality, both between countries and over time. They postulated that a high intake of sodium chloride was the common factor in Japan and elsewhere. Indeed, they suggested that the decline in stroke and stomach cancer mortality in many areas reflected the decreased use of salt as a preservative, associated with the increased use of refrigeration. It might also be pointed out that the Japanese tend to eat a highly acid diet. This is because their rice is commonly prepared using vinegar (and indeed salt) and they eat large quantities of gari, a vinegar-pickled ginger root. This is sliced thinly and used to freshen the palate between bites of sushi, to enhance its unique taste.[66]

Dietary salt use in Japan is considerably higher in the north than in the south.[67] Regional differences also occur in the incidence of stomach cancer which mirror this intake. Coggon and Acheson,[68] describing an atlas of mortality recently published for Japan, claimed that it "confirms earlier observations of high death rates [from stomach cancer] in the northwestern part of Honshu. In contrast, stomach cancer mortality is relatively low in the southern island of Kyushu."

Other inhabitants of potassium enriched volcanic islands, such as Hawaii, also display very high incidence rates for cancer of the stomach, especially if the diet is dominated by calcium poor foods such as rice. The Japanese in Hawaii, for example, have age standardized incidence rates per 100,000 per year of 34.0 for men and 15.1 for women.[69]

In contrast, one of the world's lowest age standardized incidence rates for stomach cancer is found in Senegal. Here the incidence per 100,000 per year is 3.7 for males, and 2.0 for females. Geologically, this West African country is essentially a dessicated Cretaceous and early Eocene sea. Because of this, calcium phosphate, later used in fertilizers, is the country's principal mineral product.

Given this geographical base it becomes possible to speculate about the causes of Senegal's low incidence of stomach cancer. Ledger[70] has produced a hydrological regionalization of West Africa, placing Senegal in Zone 4. That is, areas where only 1 to 3 percent of the precipitation provides runoff, the remainder being lost either into the groundwater system or to evapotranspiration. In Senegal many of the streams are very ephemeral, so groundwater plays a major role as drinking water. The mining of lime phosphate and the production of cement both indicate an abundance of subsurface calcium. Indeed, in his discussion of urban water supplies, Furon[71] cites the Senegalese as drinking water containing as much as 3.5 grams per litre of dissolved calcium and magnesium salts. In fact, the Senegalese take care to avoid water with the highest levels of magnesium because of the objectionable taste this imparts. Furon provides

Senegal as an example of exceptionally hard drinking water, possibly the world's most calcium enriched. There are no major outcrops of igneous rock or potassium enriched evaporites to add this element in quantity to the drinking water. It seems a strange coincidence that the African nation with one of the world's lowest age standardized incidence rates for stomach cancer should also drink perhaps the world's hardest water.

Particularly low age standardized mortality rates for cancer of the stomach also occur in Nicaragua, where deaths reach only 1.9 for males and 0.5 per 100,000 per year for females. Thailand also has exceptionally low age standardized death rates from this disease, 1.4 for men and 0.6 for women per 100,000 annually.[72] In both countries sedimentary rocks, especially limestones, outcrop over very large areas and, in consequence, the water is inevitably hard and probably low in potassium and sodium.

Thailand's geology, for example, is exceptionally calcareous. Much of the country's mountainous western spine consists of the massive black Thung Song limestones, which reach a thickness of over 2,450 metres. The Kaeng Krachan formation which outcrops in both the west and the rugged southeast also includes extensive Paleozoic limestones.[73] In the Eastern High Plains, a light gray crystalline Permian limestone predominates. While Mesozoic sediments, found extensively in the east, include limestone conglomerates, calcareous conglomeratic sandstones, sandy limestones and calcareous siltstones.[74] The Nicaraguan landscape is dominated by volcanoes, many of which have been active in the recent past. Masaya, for example, displayed nearly continuous volcanic activity from 1529 to 1946, while Concepcion erupted in 1963.[75] The bulk of the population, however, lives on the coastal plain, which consists largely of Tertiary clastics and limestones. Smaller outcrops of Jurassic and Cretaceous limestones and Triassic shales also occur along the western edge of Lake Nicaragua.[76]

Clearly, the soils and drinking waters of both Thailand and Nicaragua are extremely calcareous and are also probably potassium deficient. Both countries also appear likely to have selenium enriched soils. Schrauzer,[77] in a study of the relationship between selenium blood levels and breast cancer, analyzed data from 17 countries including Thailand and Costa Rica (which shares its northern border with Nicaragua). He discovered that selenium levels in female blood samples from Asia and Latin America were two to five times higher than those from Europe and the United States. In Latin America, active volcanoes are almost certainly the major source of this selenium. Thailand's selenium source is unknown. Possibly, as in the conterminous United States, this element is derived from Cretaceous shales.

137

The significance of the apparent association between both sodium and selenium and stomach cancer may also be deduced from recent changes in mortality. Coggon and Acheson,[78] for example, have shown that male incidence and mortality rates from cancer of the stomach have been falling in most countries since at least the 1950s. This is true for Japan, Chile, Finland, England, Wales, Denmark, Australia and the United States. It has been argued that improved refrigeration, food processing and handling and the declining use of nitrates may have contributed to this drop in mortality. It is also thought that butylated hydroxyanisole, a widely used food additive, may inhibit the effect of carcinogens.[79] However, it should be noted that this decline in stomach cancer has also been paralleled by a reduction in the use of sodium chloride as a preservative and by a great increase in the application of calcium rich superphosphates and triple superphosphate fertilizers by farmers. These soil additives are derived from phosphate rocks, which are particularly rich in both calcium and selenium.[80] Some support for a possible link between the greater addition of calcium and selenium to diet and declining stomach cancer mortality can be drawn from Finland. This country has experienced one of the world's most rapid drops in stomach cancer mortality, a trend which began roughly in 1950.[81] Finland is the only country in Scandinavia, and indeed one of the very few anywhere, where selenium is routinely used as a feed additive, to prevent selenium-responsive disorders in livestock.[82] This practice began at roughly the same time stomach cancer mortality started to decline.

In summary, therefore, it appears that the international evidence strongly supports a link between esophageal cancer and diets that are calcium and selenium deficient but sodium enriched. In addition, the anticipated inverse relationship between liver cancer and that of the esophagus appears to hold true in most countries. It would seem, however, that males who consume large quantities of beer may develop cancer of the liver, even in soft water areas. This may reflect the presence of carcinogens in beer, but may also be associated with the elevated levels of potassium found in this beverage.

There is some evidence to suggest that esophageal cancer and stomach cancer usually peak in the same areas. This may be because both calcium deficient drinking water and soils are generally potassium enriched. It should be noted, however, that some countries, such as Romania, display very low mortality from esophageal cancer, but have elevated stomach cancer death rates. This anomaly may reflect either the differing role played by potassium in these two cancers, or the influence of elements, such as sulphur, which were not included in this analysis.

Breast Cancer and Cancer of the Uterine Cervix

The author suggested earlier that mortality from breast cancer, in white and non-white women, in the United States can perhaps best be explained by diet and by exposure to sunlight. It was argued that this illness was associated with a diet that was rich in certain bulk and trace elements (probably, in part, from eating too much animal fat and protein), and from insufficient exposure to sunshine. The disease was also thought to be promoted by inadequate dietary selenium. If these hypotheses are correct, then global variations in the consumption of fats and proteins, exposure to solar radiation and soil selenium levels should be reflected in breast cancer incidence and mortality rates.

Epidemiologists have argued for several years that global breast cancer mortality variations are related to dietary differences. Gray, Pike and Henderson[83] demonstrated, for example, that breast cancer mortality rates are highly correlated with per capita consumption of fat (r = 0.93) and animal protein (r = 0.85). Similarly, Hirayama[84] also found that breast cancer mortality rates, in various regions of Japan, were highly correlated with fat consumption. When international breast cancer incidence rates, rather than those of mortality are compared, the relative importance of fat and animal protein is reversed, but the size of the correlation coefficients are again very high (r = 0.84 and 0.88).[85] Pike and Ross[86] concluded from this evidence that "the international correlations between per capita consumption of fat and animal protein (and certain other dietary consumption such as meat) are so high that it is not possible to confidently disentangle their separate effects."

In an effort to establish the likelihood of a strong negative worldwide correlation between solar radiation and breast cancer, this author used Pearson correlation coefficients to compare these two variables. Data on the estimated global crude rates of breast cancer incidence, per 100,000, have been published by Parkin, Stjernsward and Muir.[87] These authors subdivided the world into 24 major regions and provided best estimates for breast cancer incidence in each. Sellers[88] mapped average annual solar radiation, received on a horizontal surface at ground level, in kilolangleys per year. From his map the average annual solar radiation experienced in each of Parkin et al.'s[89] 24 regions was estimated. Correlation between crude breast cancer incidence rates and solar radiation was, therefore, possible. These two variables were found to have a marked negative correlation (r = −0.65913, p = 0.0005).

It has also been argued that selenium is a major protective agent against breast cancer. Unfortunately there is no world map of soil selenium distribution. Information is scattered and incomplete.[90] It is known, however, that the primary source of selenium is volcanic activity. It has been esti-mated that during the earth's history, volcanoes have released about 0.1 gram of selenium for every square centimetre of the earth's surface. This element is ejected in particulate form and is easily removed from volcanic gas by rain. As a consequence, selenium is usually concentrated near volcanoes. Selenium enrichment also occurs in certain sediments, such as phosphorites (18 ppm) and coals (2 ppm) but the element is generally present in very small quantities (0.05 ppm) in ultramafic igneous rocks, basalts, granites and sandstones. Shales and deep sea clays tend to con-tain intermediate levels of selenium (0.6 ppm and 0.17 ppm).[91] It would appear, therefore, that selenium is dispersed by vulcanism and by the weathering of sulphide deposits and reconcentrated biogeochemically, after which it is enriched in plant and animal tissues.[92] These processes vary with temperature and precipitation. In consequence, there is quite possibly a global gradient of soil selenium which reflects climate, with levels being highest in tropical areas. Since information about the selenium content of the world's soils is incomplete, an examination of its possible effects on cancer mortality has to be limited to the national and regional level.

One of the lowest cumulative incidence rates of breast cancer in the world is found in Senegal.[93] Here only 0.9 percent of the female popula-tion develops breast cancer by age 64. This figure rises to only 1.3 percent by age 74. For comparison, the cumulative incidence rates are 6.1 and 9.3 percent for females in the San Francisco Bay area.[94]

As has already been described, geologically speaking, Senegal is a dessicated Cretaceous and early Eocene sea gulf.[95] As a result, its major industrial activity is the mining of precipitates, lime phosphate being the principal product. Agriculture, however, occupies about 87 percent of the population, peanuts being the chief crop produced. Peanut oil mills pro-vide some 40 percent of the industrial turnover.

There may be two major reasons why breast cancer is so rare in Senegal. Peanuts are one of the best known sources of vitamin E.[96] The synergistic effects of selenium and vitamin E are well known. For reasons which are as yet unclear, the presence of vitamin E magnifies the potency of selenium.[97] High levels of vitamin E in the peanut eating diets of the inhabitants of Senegal will therefore accentuate any beneficial properties of this element. However, selenium itself is almost certainly very prevalent throughout Senegal, since calcium phosphate is one of the most seleniferous rock types known, having been shown to contain selenium levels ranging from 1 to 150 ppm, with an average content of 18 ppm.[98]

Japan also has very low cumulative incidence rates for female breast cancer. In Osaka, for example, these rates are 1.0 to age 64 and 1.4 to 74 years of age.[99] Since marine fish contain selenium in amounts that are several thousand times that found in sea water,[100] it is not surprising that a diet that is high in fish is likely to be selenium enriched. This may be especially true in Japan, where coastal waters are known to be high in selenium. Indeed, it has been claimed that Japan itself is characterized by the world's highest levels of selenium per unit area.[101] This may, or may not, be true but selenium levels are very unlikely to be low because there are some 200 volcanoes in Japan, many of them still active.[102] Sakurai and Tsuchiya[103] found, in fact, that a typical Japanese diet provided about 88 micrograms per day of selenium. For comparison, other research workers have estimated that the selenium intake in New Zealand is between 28 and 32 micrograms per day.[104] Individuals in Great Britain are thought to have an average daily consumption of 60 micrograms,[105] while those in Finland receive 30 micrograms.[106]

It would appear, therefore, that because of the volcanic origin of Japan and the major role seafood plays in its culture, dietary selenium levels are generally very high. Average size is also reduced, so increasing selenium levels per unit of body weight. Coincidentally, breast cancer rates are very low, approximately one-sixth those of the United States, Canada and certain parts of Western Europe.[107]

Soil selenium levels are known to be high in Hawaii, which is also volcanic, but so too is breast cancer mortality. This fact would, at first glance, seem to stand as a major impediment to the acceptance of the hypothesis that elevated breast cancer rates reflect, at least in part, a low selenium content in diet. However, it is interesting to note that Hawaii, with an average soil selenium content of 6 to 15 ppm, has no toxic seleniferous plants. In contrast, in parts of South Dakota and Kansas, where the soils contain less than 1 ppm selenium, toxic seleniferous plants are common.[108] This apparent anomaly is resolved when the availability, rather than the quantity, of soil selenium is examined. Elemental selenium itself is relatively stable in soils and not available to vegetation.[109] Whether it passes into plants, and hence is concentrated in the food chain, depends upon whether the soil involved is alkaline or acid.

The possible oxidation states for selenium are -2, 0, $+4$ and $+6$. Selenium in the $+6$ oxidation state (selenate) is stable in alkaline, oxidizing conditions. Soluble selenates therefore should be expected in alkaline soils and it is probably in this form that selenium uptake by plants takes place.[110] Of the compounds in which selenium is in the $+4$ oxidation state (selenite), ferric selenite is important in the environmental cycle of selenium, as it has very low solubility and absorbs on soil particles, lowering the availability of selenium to biota. Under reducing and acidic conditions, like those found in Hawaii, the formation of very insoluble elemental selenium is favored, again decreasing the availability of this element to vegetation and to animals. Mild reducing agents such as sulphur dioxide, a common volcanic gas, convert selenite to selenium. It appears that in acid soils, elemental selenium is a major 'inert' sink for selenium entering the environment. Further reduction of selenium leads to the formation of selenide. Selenides of heavy metals, such as mercury, are very insoluble indeed, explaining why when selenium and methylmercury occur together in food, neither seems to be absorbed easily by the body.[111]

This brief review of selenium's chemistry explains why crops grown in strongly acid soils, like those of Hawaii, may still possess selenium deficiencies. These occur even though the soils themselves contain large quantities of insoluble selenium. It might also be noted that the widespread use of pineapples in the Hawaiian diet probably makes many meals very acidic, so magnifying the problem of selenium insolubility.

It would appear from this review of global mortality from breast cancer that rates are depressed where diets are low in animal fats and proteins, solar radiation is high and plants and animal tissues are rich in selenates. This would explain, at least in part, why crude incidence rates for breast cancer are so low in East and Middle Africa, Middle America, Melanesia and Micronesia/Polynesia, where they are 9, 12, 14, 13 and 7 per 100,000 respectively. It would also account for the high rates experienced in North America, Northern Europe, Southern Europe and Australia and New Zealand, where they are 87, 82, 61 and 66 respectively.[112]

It has been pointed out that cancer of the uterine cervix seems to be associated with bulk and trace element deficiencies, excesses of which appear to be linked to breast cancer (Table 6,2). If this is true, then the spatial distribution of these two cancers should be reversed. From the figures presented by Parkin et al.[113] there appears some support for such a reversal. The estimated crude rate of incidence per 100,000 for cancer of the cervix is 13 in North America, while that for breast cancer is 87. In Tropical South America the relative importance of these two diseases is reversed, the incidence rate being 27 for breast cancer and 32 for cancer of the cervix. The same is true of Europe where in the north breast cancer incidence is 82 per 100,000 and that of the cervix is 17. In Southern Europe, the figures are 61 and 13 respectively, while in Eastern Europe they are 36 and 24. In Europe as a whole, therefore, breast cancer rates are generally some 3.25 times higher than those of cancer of the cervix. In contrast, in East Africa the incidence of breast cancer is estimated at 9 per 100,000 while that of the cervix is given as 21. In Middle Africa, the rates are 12 and 21 respectively, while in Northern Africa they are 25 and 19. Cancer of the cervix is more common than breast cancer in West Africa. This is also true of Southern Africa where the incidence of cancer of the cervix is 27 and of the breast 20. In Africa as

142

a whole, therefore, the incidence of cancer of the cervix is 1.36 times higher than that of breast cancer, giving support to the argument that it is associated with bulk and trace element deficiencies.

Where mortality from cancer of the breast and cervix have been mapped in great detail, this relationship can be examined more precisely. This is the case in England and Wales, where 1,366 local authorities were used as the basis for mapping.[114] As can be seen from Figure 8,4 there is no overlap between local authorities with standardized mortality ratios that are significantly low, in the bottom tenth of the distribution, for cancer of the breast and of the cervix. That is, there is no local authority in England and Wales that has a significantly low, tenth decile death rate for both illnesses. When local authorities with standardized mortality ratios that are significantly high, in the top tenth, for both diseases are mapped, there is only one local authority that has an elevated death rate for both cancer of the breast and of the cervix (Figure 7,4). However, this is Stone Rural District, the one authority that the authors of the *Atlas of Cancer Mortality in England and Wales 1968-78* claim should be ignored because of the unreliability of its mortality data. This occurs because there is a terminal care hospital for cancer patients in Stone, and this local authority is often recorded as the place of death for individuals who, in fact, originally resided elsewhere. This practice naturally renders the data for this particular local authority virtually worthless. This author, therefore, feels justified in ignoring this one area of overlap. The probability that there would be no meaningful overlap on either map (Figure 7,4 and Figure 8,4) was calculated to be approximately 0.08. That is, there are only eight chances in one hundred that these distributions could be due to chance alone. From the author's point of view what makes this reversal more convincing is that he did not notice it until it had been predicted by the analysis illustrated in Table 6,2. In summary, therefore, where the most detailed mortality mapping has been carried out, the postulated inverse relationship between breast cancer and that of the cervix is found to hold true.

Melanoma

It has been shown that whites in the United States appear to develop melanoma when iodine intake is high yet diet is deficient in most other major bulk and trace elements (Table 9,2). When this happens, exposure to strong sunlight, in non-pigmented races, appears to be associated with high melanoma mortality.

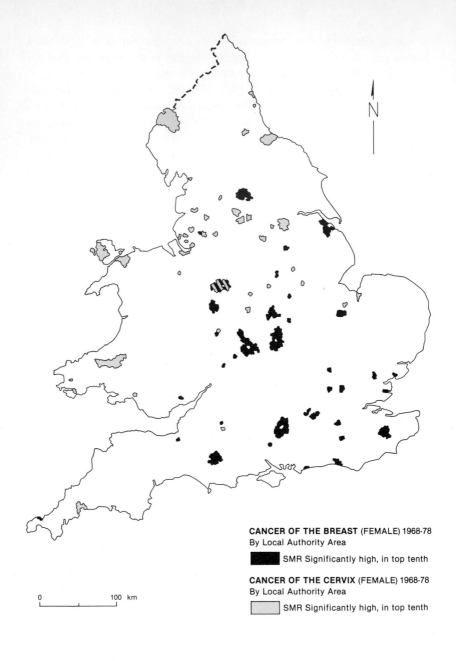

CANCER OF THE BREAST (FEMALE) 1968-78
By Local Authority Area

▇ SMR Significantly high, in top tenth

CANCER OF THE CERVIX (FEMALE) 1968-78
By Local Authority Area

▨ SMR Significantly high, in top tenth

0   100 km

Figure 7,4   A Comparison of Significantly High Mortality from Cancer of the Breast
and Uterine Cervix in England and Wales (1968-1978)

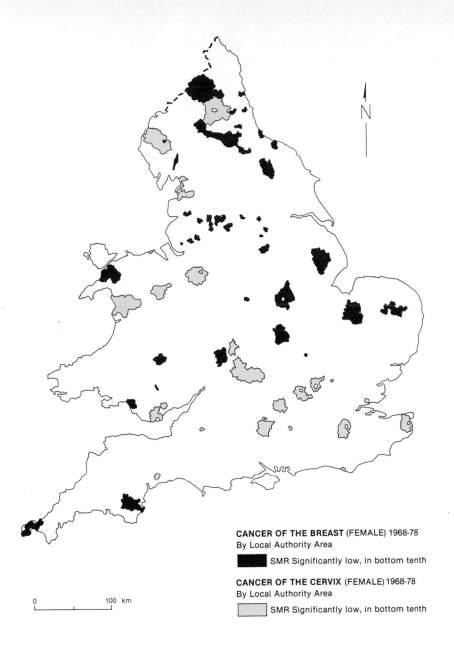

CANCER OF THE BREAST (FEMALE) 1968-78
By Local Authority Area

■ SMR Significantly low, in bottom tenth

CANCER OF THE CERVIX (FEMALE) 1968-78
By Local Authority Area

▢ SMR Significantly low, in bottom tenth

0   100 km

Figure 8,4   A Comparison of Significantly Low Mortality from Cancer of the Breast
and Uterine Cervix in England and Wales (1968-1978)

145

This relationship appears to explain why the world's highest levels of malignant melanoma are found in Queensland, Australia, where the incidence per 100,000 is nearly 40.[115] Australia is a continent dominated by low soil levels of a variety of bulk and trace elements, because there has been "no recent mountain building, little recent vulcanism outside the Western District of Victoria and no ice age to remove the old soils and start new ones on their way."[116] In consequence, "the recurring theme of Australia soils is old age and poverty."[117] Indeed, "we have told one another, to the point of weariness that Australian soils are naturally deficient in phosphorus."[118] Other trace elements known to be relatively lacking from Australian soils include molybdenum, zinc, potassium and calcium.[119] However, the amount of salt in the subcontinent's soils varies greatly. Along the humid coast of Queensland, where melanoma levels are highest, heavy rainfall produces leaching and podsolized soils are widely developed. These soils are acidic and usually of poor natural fertility.[120] Inland, rainfall is lower, as is melanoma incidence. Here, however, black earths predominate. These soils are amongst the most fertile in Australia and often contain high levels of phosphorus.[121] In addition, farther east, in areas of even lower rainfall, solonized soils, particularly mallee soils, are very common and these characteristically have a very high sodium chloride content.[122] In summary, therefore, the soils of coastal Queensland, where melanoma rates are highest, are leached by heavy rainfall and are deficient in a wide variety of bulk and trace elements. Farther inland, levels of phosphorus and sodium chloride rise, as precipitation levels fall. Mirroring this rise in bulk and trace elements is a decline in melanoma.

It would appear, however, that for melanoma to occur, not only must diet be deficient in a variety of bulk and trace elements, it must also be iodine enriched (Table 9,2). It is believed by geologists that the primary source of the world's iodine is the weathering of igneous rocks. Countries such as Switzerland, Norway, Sweden and Finland, therefore, are likely to have many iodine enriched soils because of their bedrock geology.[123] Where these are also deficient in bulk and trace elements, such as phosphorus, magnesium, sodium and zinc, then melanoma might be expected to be prevalent.

Iodine, released from igneous rocks by weathering, enters rivers in solution and eventually reaches the sea, therefore the oceans have become great reservoirs, containing some 25 percent of the earth's total iodine.[124] It is believed that some of the ocean's iodine enters the atmosphere in a gaseous state, or is absorbed onto dust particles and then is returned by precipitation to the land.[125] As a result of this process, the oldest soils tend to be the richest in iodine, while newer soils have had insufficient time to develop such high concentrations. This is perhaps why the soils of the southern United States are rich in iodine. The same is true of unglaciated southern England and Queensland, all areas where melanoma is prevalent.

It is known that iodine enrichment is most common along the coasts. Beeson,[126] for example, has estimated that between 22 and 50 micrograms of iodine per acre fall from the atmosphere each year onto the Atlantic Coastal Plain, while only 0.7 micrograms are deposited in the Great Lakes region. Indeed, it seems likely that in coastal areas iodine may be directly absorbed from the air by residents.[127] This process explains why goitre occurs in the interiors of all continents but not on the coasts. It would appear, therefore, that the high melanoma mortality of Queensland is probably associated with soils which are, as expected, enriched in iodine but deficient in most other bulk and trace elements.

The world's lowest incidence of malignant melanoma occurs in parts of Japan, where the annual rate is 0.2 cases per 100,000. This level is less than one percent of that of Queensland.[128] Since melanoma appears to be associated with high soil iodine levels, it is perhaps surprising to discover that this disease is so rare in Japan, where soils tend to be iodine enriched. However, Japanese diets are not usually deficient in other bulk and trace elements. Indeed, because of their highly salted cuisine, the Japanese have what is probably one of the world's highest intakes of sodium chloride ($\geqslant 15$ g NaCl/day).[129] Other groups that also have unusual dietary habits and depressed melanoma mortality rates include the Jews of Israel and the whites of Hawaii. Breast cancer, in contrast, appears to be associated with bulk and trace element excesses and underexposure to the sun, that is with the reverse of many of the factors associated with melanoma. It is of interest to note, therefore, that the white female population of Hawaii, which despite a predilection for sunbathing, has such a low melanoma mortality rate,[131] experiences one of the world's highest breast cancer mortalities.[132] A similar reversal of the two specific cancer types can be seen throughout the conterminous United States (Figure 3,1). In contrast, Japanese women have low mortality from both diseases, perhaps because high dietary selenium levels give protection against breast cancer, even if salt is consumed to excess. The Japanese, however, also eat relatively little meat, so reducing the risk of breast cancer.[133]

It should be pointed out that since melanoma appears related, at least in part, to iodine excess, it is very unlikely to be prevalent in those regions that suffer high levels of thyroid disturbances, such as goitre. This is certainly the case in the United States (Figure 9,4).[134]

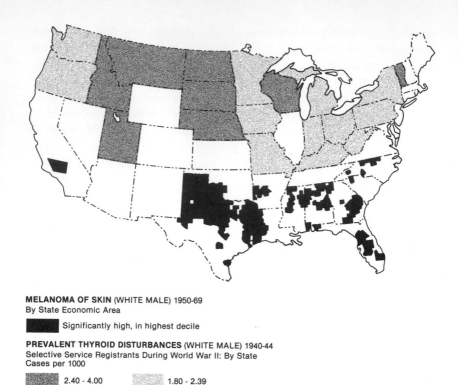

MELANOMA OF SKIN (WHITE MALE) 1950-69
By State Economic Area

■ Significantly high, in highest decile

PREVALENT THYROID DISTURBANCES (WHITE MALE) 1940-44
Selective Service Registrants During World War II: By State
Cases per 1000

▓ 2.40 - 4.00   ░ 1.80 - 2.39

Figure 9,4 A Comparison, in the United States, of the Distribution of Total Thyroid
Disturbances Among White Male Selective Service Registrants During
World War II and White Male Mortality from Melanoma (1950-1969)

THE ROLE OF DRINKING WATER

It can be seen from the preceding analyses that drinking water supply appears to be extremely significant in determining the distribution of mortality
from specific cancers. This may be because the presence, or absence, of
bulk and trace elements in potable water is relatively constant. As a consequence, individuals drinking or cooking with such supplies are exposed
repeatedly to the same excesses or deficiencies. Of course, the chemical
composition of such drinking water, in turn, reflects the geology of the
drainage basins and aquifers from which it is derived and the treatment to
which it is subjected before delivery. Indeed, even the nature of the pipes
carrying potable water can influence its final quality.

The role played by geology, through drinking water and soils, can be best
illustrated in England and Wales, where Gardner[135] identified those local

148

authorities that had the largest number of high, or low, standardized mortality ratios, from 23 and 21 major types of specific cancers, in both sexes. These were essentially the cancer "black" and "bright" spots. All local authorities with seven or more occurrences of a specific cancer, that was significantly high and in the top tenth of the distribution, were identified. So, too, were all local authority areas with five or more occurrences of cancer that were significantly low, and in the bottom tenth of the distribution. This analysis yielded seven local authorities that were particularly badly affected by permutations of cancer of the esophagus, stomach, large intestine, rectum, pancreas, lung, breast, cervix, other uterus, ovary, bladder, prostate and pleural mesothelioma.

When these seven administrative bodies are located, on the geological map of England and Wales, it is found that four are situated in areas of Bunter Sandstone. These include Kirby Urban District, Huyton-with-Roby Urban District and Widnes Municipal Borough, all of which are in Lancashire. In addition, two of the remaining three are situated on the Productive Coal Measures, namely Jarrow Municipal Borough in Durham and Longbenton Urban District in Northumberland. Even more interesting is the fact that Stone Rural District, Staffordshire which has almost twice as many high specific cancer rates as any other local authority in England and Wales, lies on the unconformity between the Bunter Sandstone, Keuper Marls and the Barren Upper Coal Measures. This is one of the very few locations in Britain where the Bunter Sandstones and Coal Measures meet unconformably. The water served to consumers in Stone is quite saline, with a maximum sodium content of 56 ppm and a mean concentration of 38 ppm. It has the highest sodium levels of any water supplied by the Upper Trent Division of the Severn-Trent Water Authority.[136] The author realizes, however, that cancer mortality in Stone Rural District has been exaggerated by the presence of a terminal care hospital for cancer patients of all ages, in a district of relatively small population. Nevertheless, this facility presumably serves the surrounding local authority areas. To summarize, then, although the Bunter Sandstones and the Productive Coal Measures outcrop over only 5.7 percent and 5.0 percent in England and Wales respectively,[137] they are associated with 85.7 percent of the most cancer-prone local authorities in these two countries.

Wells and Kirkaldy[138] have described the Bunter Sandstones as all-important to the water supply of the English Midlands. The amount of water which is stored in any aquifer reflects both its volume and the pore space available. Since the area covered by the coarse grained Bunter Sandstone is some 5.7 percent of England and Wales, it holds enormous quantities of water. Particularly where covered by Keuper Marl, it is a natural underground reservoir which is tapped by countless wells. The water is relatively soft and suitable for use in the brewing industry: Burton-on-Trent being dependent on this fact for its prosperity.[139]

149

The Bunter and Keuper Sandstones appear to have originated as barchans (sand dunes) in a Permo-Triassic desert and pass laterally into mudflats, with salt deposits which occupy the former site of the Zechstein Sea.[140] The Keuper consists of three major rock types: sandstones, so-called marls and mineral salts. The marls reach a thickness of some 915 metres under the Cheshire Plain and are interpreted by geologists as an ancient loessic deposit.[141] Similar wind-blown sediments occurring at the surface today throughout much of eastern Iran, the Kazakhstan, Afghanistan and the People's Republic of China are associated with the world's highest levels of esophageal cancer, a relationship that has been discussed elsewhere.

Mineral salts are found in the Keuper in both western and eastern England, but differ markedly in chemical composition. In eastern England the evaporation of the Keuper "lakes" deposited large volumes of gypsum, that is hydrated calcium sulphate, which occurs near the surface in Nottinghamshire, Leicestershire and Derbyshire. Apart from carbonates, gypsum, rich in calcum, is the first of the mineral salts to be deposited from a salt lake or inland sea that is undergoing rapid evaporation.[142] A later stage of desiccation results in the deposition of rock salt (sodium chloride) which is found, and in some cases mined, in the Keuper of western England, in Lancashire, Cheshire, Staffordshire, Worcester and Somerset.[143]

It is of interest to note that 57 percent of the most cancer prone areas of England and Wales are located in the west, where most of the drinking water is drawn from ancient saline loess. In contrast, local authorities situated on the Bunter and Keuper of eastern England, where the sediments are rich in hydrated calcium sulphate, do not suffer elevated cancer mortalities.[144]

Elevated cancer mortality in the London borough of Barking may be associated with high levels of sodium and strontium in drinking water supplies. Water has been abstracted from aquifers in this area for many years. However, as groundwater abstraction from the London Basin's confined aquifer and along the lower reaches of the Thames increased, the natural hydraulic gradient reversed, allowing saline intrusion. Estuarine river water, therefore, flowed into the London Tertiaries and into the Chalk, wherever these aquifers were in hydraulic continuity with the Thames. As a result, the chlorine concentrations are particularly high, in the order of 1,000 ppm, in groundwater beneath certain parts of eastern London, including Barking.[145] In addition, the strontium to calcium ratio of chalk groundwater below the London Clay is 1:13, which must be considered extremely high when compared with the average of 1:670 for carbonate sediments in general. This element is thought to be derived from the strontium enriched microfossils that comprise an appreciable part of the chalk.[146] Indeed, the most mineralized water the author has been able to discover anywhere in England and Wales is taken from boreholes in the

Dagenham area, by the Essex Water Company. Raw water in this region has a total hardness of 535 ppm, and includes 280 ppm calcium, 260 ppm magnesium, 185 ppm sodium, 14.3 ppm potassium and 309 ppm chloride. It has a pH value of 7.2.[147]

Gardner's[148] list of cancer "bright spots" also appears to reflect the influence of bedrock geology. Of the 12 local authorities identified, 10 are located in areas of Magnesium Limestone, the eastern facies (hydrated calcium sulphate) of the Keuper Marl, the Middle and Upper Lias, the Great Oolite or the Cretaceous Chalk. All these deposits are highly calcareous, reflecting the presence of either limestones, or chalk, or of lake evaporites such as gypsum. Collectively these lithologies cover less than 23 percent of England and Wales, but are the sites of 83 percent of its least cancer prone local authorities. This distribution occurs despite the fact that these lowland areas support the bulk of agriculture and industry. Water derived from chalk aquifers can be very calcium rich indeed. The Southern Water Authority draws much of its water from this lithology. At the Andover pumping station, this has a mean calcium content of 264 ppm, yet only contains 8 ppm of magnesium. Similarly, the Winchester pumping station draws water from the chalk that has a mean calcium content of 258 ppm, yet has only 10 ppm magnesium, 7.9 ppm sodium and 0.98 ppm potassium.[149]

The two remaining local authorities on the "bright spot" list, Carmathen and Llandeilo Rural Districts, contain almost the entire extent of the Llandeilo in Britain. This consists of an enormous thickness of Ordovician limestones, rapidly alternating with thin sandstones and flags. The Llandeilo also includes a volcanic ash deposit that may be rich in selenium.[150]

In summary, therefore, the author is forced to conclude that the maps of cancer mortality in England and Wales reflect, in part at least, the chemical composition of drinking water. This in turn is controlled by the geology of the drainage basins and aquifers from which it is derived. An interesting example of this apparent relationship can be seen in Cornwall where cancer of the esophagus is particularly common in women. Standardized mortality ratios are significantly high, in the top tenth, for West Penwith, Kerrier, Newquay and Liskeard, for females and in Wodebridge and Padstow for men.[151] As might be anticipated from Table 2,2, calcium levels in surface sediments are amongst the lowest in England.[152] This is reflected in the hardness and calcium content of the water supplied by South West Water to Penwith District Council, which has an average carbonate hardness of 25 ppm and contains 18.7 ppm of calcium. The figures for that used in Kerrier District Council are 28.2 ppm and 19.8 ppm respectively.[153]

REFERENCES

1. PARKIN, D.M., STJERNSWARD, J. and MUIR, C.S., "Estimates of the Worldwide Frequency of Twelve Major Cancers", *Bulletin of the World Health Organization* ,vol. 62(2), 1984, pp. 163-182.

2. GREER, J.S., MADAUS, J.H. and MAUSTELLER, J.W., "Potassium", *Encyclopedia of Chemical Technology*, vol. 18. New York: John Wiley, 1982, p. 912.

3. DANCY, W.B., "Potassium Compounds", *Encyclopedia of Chemical Technology*, vol. 18. New York: John Wiley, 1982, p. 921.

4. DAY, N.E., "Cancer of the Oesophagus", *British Medical Bulletin*, vol. 40(4), 1984, pp. 329-334.

5. COGGAN, D. and ACHESON, E.D., "Cancer of the Stomach", *British Medical Bulletin*, vol. 40(4), 1984, pp. 335-341.

6. COOK-MOZAFFARI, P. and VAN RENSBURG, S., "Cancer of the Liver", *British Medical Bulletin*, vol. 40(4), 1984, pp. 342-345.

7. DAY, *op. cit.*, p. 329.

8. COGGAN and ACHESON, *op. cit.*, pp. 335-336.

9. COOK-MOZAFFARI and VAN RENSBURG, *op. cit.*, p. 342.

10. *Ibid.*

11. SCHAPERA, I. and GOODWIN, A.J.H., "Work and Wealth", in SCHAPERA, I. (ed.), *The Bantu-Speaking Tribes of South Africa: An Ethnographical Survey*. London: Routledge and Kegan Paul, 1962, p. 133. Part of this quotation is taken from STAYT, H.A., *The BaVenda*. Oxford: University Press, 1931, p. 48.

12. CHINA MAP PRESS, *Atlas of Cancer Mortality in the People's Republic of China*. Beijing: China Map Press, 1979, pp. 23-24 and 31-32.

13. GARDNER, M.J., WINTER, P.D., TAYLOR, C.P. and ACHESON, E.D., *Atlas of Cancer Mortality in England and Wales 1968-78*. Chichester: Wiley, 1983.

14. GARDNER, M.J., "Mapping Cancer Mortality in England and Wales", *British Medical Bulletin*, vol. 40(4), 1984, pp. 320-328.

15. *Ibid.*, plate 1.

16. UNWIN, D., *Introductory Spatial Analysis*. London: Methuen, 1981, pp. 30-66.

17. GARDNER, *et al.*, *op. cit.*, plate III.

18. GEOLOGICAL SURVEY, *Geological Map of Great Britain: Sheet 2, England and Wales*, 2nd Edition, 1957. Scale 1:625,000.

19. GARDNER, *et al.*, *op. cit.*

20. IMPERIAL COLLEGE OF SCIENCE AND TECHNOLOGY, APPLIED GEOCHEMISTRY RESEARCH GROUP, *The Wolfson Geochemical Atlas of England and Wales*. Oxford: University Press, 1978, pp. 28-29.

21. GEOLOGICAL SURVEY, *op. cit.*

22. PITTY, A.F., *Introduction to Geomorphology*. London: Methuen, 1971, p. 188.

23. DEGRÉMONT, G., *Water Treatment Handbook*. English edition. New York: Taylor and Carlisle, 1973, p. 1086.

24. SEVERN-TRENT WATER AUTHORITY, *Reports and Accounts 1978-1979*. Birmingham: 1979, p. 14.

25. CITY OF MANCHESTER, *The Water-Supply Undertaking of the City of Manchester*. Manchester: 1974, 32 pp.

26. YORKSHIRE WATER AUTHORITY, *Annual Report and Accounts for the Year Ending 31st March 1978*. 1978, p. 10.

27. IMPERIAL COLLEGE OF SCIENCE AND TECHNOLOGY, *op. cit.*

28. WELSH NATIONAL WATER DEVELOPMENT AUTHORITY, *First Annual Report for the Period Ending 31st March 1975.* Brecon, Powys: 1975, 10:11:2 Water Quality Data Tables 1-19.

29. THAMES CONSERVANCY, *Water Resources Act 1963. Section 14 Report of Survey 1969: Thames Catchment Area and London Excluded Area. London: 1969, p. 47, and Table XIX.*

30. DAY, *op. cit.*, p. 332.

31. *Ibid.*

32. BUREAU DE RECHERCHES GÉOLOGIQUES ET MINIÈRES SERVICE GÉOLOGIQUE NATIONAL, Cartes des Eaux Minérales et Thermales de la France, 1973. Scale 1:1,000,000.

33. DAY, *op. cit.*, pp. 332-333.

34. *Ibid.*

35. DAINELLI, G., *Atlante Fisico Economico d'Italia.* Costituzione Litologica, Scale 1:2,500,000. Milano: Consociazione Turistica Italiana, MCMXL (1940).

36. MINISTERSTVO GEOLOGIII I OKHRANY NEDR SSSR, *Geologiehiskaya Karta SSSR.* Scale 1:2,500,000. Chief editor Glavnyy Redaktor, D.V. Nalivkin, 1956, and CHINESE PETROLEUM CORPORATION, *Geologic Map of the Republic of China.* Supervised by Chao-yi Meng. Scale 1:4,000,000. 1970.

37. CHORLEY, R.J., SCHUMM, S.A. and SUGDEN, D.E., *Geomorphology.* London: Methuen, 1984, pp. 411 and 563-566.

38. DAY, *op. cit.*, pp. 329-331.

39. PAVELKO, I.M. and TARASOV, M.N., "Hydrochemical Maps of the Rivers of Kazakhstan and Their Use for the Rapid Forecasting of the Mineralization and Ion Composition of Waters of Prospective Reservoirs", *Soviet Hydrology: Selected Papers,* vol. 6, 1967, pp. 495-508.

40. *Ibid.*, pp. 505-507.

41. GARDNER, J.S., *Physical Geography*. New York: Harper's College Press, 1977, pp. 407 and 516.

42. PAVELKO and TARASOV, *op. cit.*

43. KMET, J. and MAHBOUBI, E., "Esophageal Cancer in the Caspian Littoral of Iran", *Science*, vol. 175, 1972, pp. 846-853.

44. PARKIN, *et al.*, *op. cit.*, p. 169 and DAY, *op. cit.*, pp. 329-330.

45. DAY, *op. cit.*, p. 329.

46. *Ibid.*, pp. 329-330.

47. CHINA MAP PRESS, *op. cit.*, pp. 23-24 and 31-32.

48. MENG, *op. cit.*

49. *Ibid.*

50. HSIEH, CHIAO-MIN, *Atlas of China*, SALTER, C.L. (ed.). New York: McGraw-Hill, 1973, p. 48.

51. DAY, *op. cit.*, p. 329.

52. DEPARTMENTS OF GEOLOGICAL SURVEY OF NORTHERN RHODESIA, SOUTHERN RHODESIA AND NYASALAND, *Provisional Geological Map of the Federation of Rhodesia and Nyasaland*, 1960. Scale 1:2,500,000.

53. LAUBSCHER, J.F., *Sex, Custom and Psychopathology: A Study of South African Pagan Natives*. New York: Humanities Press, 1952, pp. 82-84.

54. SCHAPERA, *et al.*, *op. cit.*, pp. 132-133, and LESTRADE, G.P., "Domestic and Cultural Life", in SCHAPERA, *op. cit.*, pp. 125-126.

55. DAY, *op. cit.*, p. 329.

56. LATHAM, P., *Romania: A Complete Guide*. London: The Garnstone Press, 1967, 245 pp.

57. *Ibid.*, and MATLEY, I.M., *Romania: A Profile*. New York: Praeger, 1970, 292 pp.

58. LATHAM, *op. cit.*

59. *Ibid.*

60. COGGAN, *et al.*, *op. cit.*, p. 335.

61. SCHROEDER, H.A., "Municipal Drinking Water and Cardiovascular Death-Rates", *Journal of the American Medical Association*, vol. 195, 1966, pp. 125-129.

62. BRICKLIN, M. and CLAESSENS, S., *The Natural Healing Cookbook*. Emmaus, Pa.: Rodale Press, 1981, pp. 297-298.

63. JOOSEENS, J.C. and GEBOERS, J., "Salt and Hypertension", *Preventive Medicine*, vol. 12, 1983, pp. 53-59.

64. TOHYAMA, H., *Quick and Easy Sushi: Cook Book*. Tokyo: Joie, 1983, 108 pp.

65. JOOSSENS and GEBOERS, *op. cit.*

66. TOHYAMA, *op. cit.* ,p. 104.

67. DAHL, L.K., "Salt Intake and Hypertension", in GENEST, J., KOIW, E. and KVECHEL, O. (eds.), *Hypertension: Physiopathology and Treatment*. New York: McGraw-Hill, 1977, pp. 548-559.

68. COGGAN, *et al.*, *op. cit.*, pp. 336-337.

69. *Ibid.*, p. 335.

70. LEDGER, D.C., "Some Hydrological Characteristics of West African Rivers", *Transactions, Institute of British Geographers*, vol. 35, 1964, pp. 73-90.

71. FURON, R., *The Problem of Water: A World Study*. English edition. London: Faber and Faber, 1967, p. 80.

72. SERGI, M. (in collaboration with HATTORI, H., NOYE, H., and SERGI, R.), *Age-Adjusted Death Rates for Cancer for Selected Sites (A −* classification) in 40 Countries in 1976. Nagoya: Sergi Institute for Cancer Epidemiology, 1981. Cited in COGGAN, *et al., op. cit.*, p. 336.

73. STERNSTEIN, L., *Thailand: The Environment of Modernization.* Sydney: McGraw-Hill, 1976, pp. 20-23, 200 pp.

74. *Ibid.*

75. MacDONALD, G.A., *Volcanoes.* Englewood Cliffs, N.J.: Prentice-Hall, 1972, pp. 442-443, 510 pp.

76. HEALY, P.F., *Archaeology of the Rivas Region: Nicaragua.* Waterloo: Wilfrid Laurier, 1980, pp. 10-11, 382 pp.

77. SCHRAUZER cited by BRICKLIN, *et al., op. cit.*, pp. 225-226.

78. COGGAN, *et al., op. cit.*, p. 337.

79. ROSS, W.S., "At Last, an Anti-Cancer Diet", *Reader's Digest*, vol. 122(733), 1983, pp. 49-53.

80. KELLER, E.A., *Environmental Geology.* 2nd Edition. Columbus: Charles E. Merrill, 1979, p. 328-329.

81. COGGAN, *et al., op. cit.*

82. NORRMAN, E., *Selebrist*, in VÅR NÄRING, 2/1977. Cited by SCHALIN, G., "Multiple Sclerosis and Selenium", in LÅG, J. (ed.), *Geomedical Aspects of Present and Future Research.* Oslo: The Norwegian Academy of Science and Letters, 1980, p. 95.

83. GRAY, G.E., PIKE, M.C. and HENDERSON, B.E., "Breast Cancer Incidence and Mortality Rates in Different Countries in Relation to Known Risk Factors and Dietary Practices", *British Journal of Cancer*, vol. 39, 1979, pp. 1-7.

84. HIRAYAMA, R., "Epidemiology of Breast Cancer with Special Reference to the Role of Diet", *Preventive Medicine*, vol. 7, 1978, pp. 173-195.

85. GRAY, *et al.* (1979), *op. cit.*, pp. 1-7.

86. PIKE, M.C. and ROSS, R.K., "Breast Cancer", *British Medical Bulletin*, vol. 40(4), 1984, p. 352.

87. PARKIN, *et al.*, *op. cit.*

88. SELLERS, W.D., *Physical Climatology*. Chicago: University of Chicago Press, 1965, p. 25.

89. PARKIN, *et al.*, *op. cit.*

90 SUBCOMMITTEE OF SELENIUM, Committee on Animal Nutrition, Board of Agriculture, National Research Council, *Selenium in Nutrition*. Revised edition. Washington, D.C.: National Academy Press, 1983, pp. 73-74.

91. FLEISCHER, M., cited by KELLER, E.A., *op. cit.*, pp. 328-329.

92. SUBCOMMITTEE ON SELENIUM, *op. cit.*, pp. 3-39.

93. PIKE and ROSS, *op. cit.*, p. 351.

94. *Ibid.*

95. ENCYCLOPEDIA BRITANNICA, "Senegal", vol. 20. Chicago: William Benton, 1972, p. 217.

96. BRICKLIN, *et al.*, *op. cit.*, pp. 16-17.

97. SUBCOMMITTEE ON SELENIUM, *op. cit.*, pp. 51-56.

98. FLEISCHER, *op. cit.*

99. PIKE and ROSS, *op. cit.*, p. 351.

100. MORRIS, V.C. and LEVANDER, O.A., "Selenium Content of Foods", *Journal of Nutrition*, vol. 100, 1970, pp. 1383-1388.

101. JANSOON, B., MALAHY, M.A. and SEIBERT, G.B., *Geographical Distribution of Gastrointestinal Cancer and Breast Cancer and its Relation to Selenium Deficiency*. National Large Bowel Cancer Project, University of Texas System Cancer Center, M.D. Anderson Hospital and Tumor Institute, Houston, Texas, 1976.

102. MacDONALD, *op. cit.*, pp. 442-443.

103. SAKURAI, H. and TSUCHIYA, K., "A Tentative Recommendation for Maximum Daily Intake of Selenium", *Environ. Physiol. Biochem.*, vol. 5, 1975, pp. 107-118.

104. THOMSON, C.D. and ROBINSON, M.F., "Selenium in Human Health and Disease with Emphasis on those Aspects Peculiar to New Zealand", *Americal Journal of Clinical Nutrition*, vol. 33, 1980, pp. 303-323.

105. THORN, J., ROBERTSON, J., BUSS, D.H. and BUNTON, N.G., "Trace Nutrients. Selenium in British Foods", *British Journal of Nutrition*, vol. 39, 1978, p. 391.

106. KOIVISTOINEN P., "Mineral Composition of Finnish Foods: N, K, Ca, Mg, P, S, Fe, Cu, Mn, Zn, Mo, Co, Ni, Cr, F, Se, Si, Rb, Al, B, Br, Hg, As, Cd, Pb and Ash", *Acta Agric. Scand.*, Supplement 22, 1980, p. 171.

107. PIKE and ROSS, *op. cit.*, p. 351.

108. KELLER, *op. cit.*, p. 339.

109. *Ibid.*

110. DEMAYO, A., TAYLOR, M.C. and REEDER, S.W., *Guidelines for Surface Water Quality. Vol. 1 - Inorganic Chemical Substances: Selenium.* Inland Waters Directorate, Water Quality Branch, Ottawa, Canada, 1979, pp. 2-3.

111. *Ibid.*

112. PARKIN, *et al.*, *op. cit.*

113. *Ibid.*

114. GARDNER, *op. cit.*, p. 320.

115. GREEN, A., "Incidence and Reporting of Cutaneous Melanoma in Queensland", *Australian Journal of Dermatology*, vol. 23, 1982, pp. 105-109.

116. LEEPER, G.W., "Soils", in LEEPER, G.W. (ed.), *The Australian Environment*. 4th Edition. CSIRO, Victoria: Melbourne University Press, 1970, pp. 21-31.

117. *Ibid.*, p. 22.

118. *Ibid.*

119. *Ibid.*, p. 23.

120. ROBINSON, K.W., *Australia, New Zealand and the South West Pacific: A Systematic Regional Geography*. London: University of London Press, 1962, pp. 41-45.

121. HUBBLE, G.D., "Soils", in MOORE, R.M. (ed.), *Australian Grasslands*. Canberra: Australian National University Press, 1970, pp. 44-58.

122. *Ibid.*

123. RANKAMA, K. and SAHAMA, T.G., *Geochemistry*. Chicago: Chicago University Press, 1955, 912 pp. *See also* KELLER, *op. cit.*, pp. 334-337.

124. SHACKELLETE, H.T. and CUTHBERT, M.E., "Iodine Content of Plant Groups as Influenced by Variations in Rock and Soil Type", in CANNON, H.L. and DAVIDSON, D.F. (eds.), *Relations of Geology and Trace Elements to Nutrition*. Geological Society of American Special Paper 90, 1967, pp. 31-45.

125. KELLER, *op. cit.*, pp. 334-337.

126. BEESON, K.C., "The Relation of Soil to Micronutrient Element Content of Plants and to Animal Nutrition", in LAMB, C.A., BENTLEY, O.G. and BEATTIE, C., (eds.), *Trace Elements*. New York: Academy Press, 1958, 410 pp.

127. VOUGHT, R.L., LONDON, W.T. and BROWN, F.A., "Note on Atmosphere Iodine and its Absorption in Man", in CANNON, H. and DAVIDSON, D.F., (eds.), *Relation to Geology and Trace Elements to Nutrition*. Geological Society of America Special Paper 90, 1967, p. 11.

128. ARMSTRONG, B.K., "Melanoma of the Skin", *British Medical Bulletin*, vol. 40(4), 1984, p. 346.

129. JOOSSENS and GEBOERS, *op. cit.*, pp. 53-59.

130. ARMSTRONG, *op. cit.*, p. 348.

131. *Ibid.*, p. 347.

132. PIKE, *et al.*, *op. cit.*, p. 351.

133. KIRSCHMANN, J.D. and DUNNE, L.J., *Nutrition Almanac.* 2nd Edition. New York: McGraw-Hill, 1984, 313 pp.

134. STRAIN, W.H., PORIES, W.J., MANSOUR, E.G., and FLYNN, A., "Therapies for Environmental Element Deficiencies and Toxic Excesses", in FREEDMAN, J., (ed.), *Trace Element Geochemistry in Health and Disease.* The Geological Society of America, Special Paper 155, 1975, pp. 91-97. See also MASON, J.T., McKAY, F.W., HOOVER, R., BLOT, W.J. and FRAUMENI, J.F. Jr., *Atlas of Cancer Mortality for U.S. Counties: 1950-1969.* DHEW Publication No. (NIH) 75-780, U.S. Department of Health, Education and Welfare, 1975.

135. GARDNER, M.J., "Mapping Cancer Mortality in England and Wales", *British Medical Bulletin*, vol. 40(4), 1984, pp. 322-323.

136. SEVERN-TRENT WATER AUTHORITY, *Water Quality 1983/84 Appendix 7 — Upper Trent Division.* Birmingham: Severn-Trent Water, 1984.

137. GEOLOGICAL SURVEY, *Geological Map of Great Britain: Sheet 2, England and Wales.* 2nd Edition. 1957. Scale 1:625,000.

138. WELLS, A.K. and KIRKALDY, J.F., *Outline of Historical Geology.* London: Thomas Murby, 1959, p. 226.

139. *Ibid.*

140. *Ibid.*, pp. 224-231.

141. *Ibid.*, p. 227.

142. *Ibid.*, p. 228.

143. *Ibid.*

144. GARDNER, *op. cit.*, p. 323.

145. WATER RESOURCES BOARD, *The Hydrogeology of the London Basin.* Reading: Reading Bridge House, 1972, pp. 107-110.

146. *Ibid.*, p. 136.

147. ESSEX WATER COMPANY, WATER QUALITY DEPARTMENT, *Annual Statistics 1984 (January - December).* Romford, Essex. Tables 5-6.

148. GARDNER, *op. cit.*, p. 323.

149. SOUTHERN WATER AUTHORITY, Hampshire Division Process Laboratory. Laboratory Data Handling System. *Interrogation Summary Report*, 31/10/1985. Computer printout supplied by R.W. Brett.

150. WELLS and KIRKALDY, *op. cit.*, pp. 36-38.

151. GARDNER, M.J., WINTER, P.D., TAYLOR, C.P. and ACHESON, E.D., *Atlas of Cancer Mortality in England and Wales 1968-1978.* Chichester: Wiley, 1983, pp. 12-13.

152. IMPERIAL COLLEGE OF SCIENCE AND TECHNOLOGY AP-PLIED GEOCHEMISTRY RESEARCH GROUP, *The Wolfson Geochemical Atlas of England and Wales.* Oxford: Oxford University Press, 1978, maps 28 and 29.

153. CHAVE, P.A., Scientific Service Manager, South West Water Authority, personal communication 18/11/1985.

*We have, I hope, abandoned the convenient
but restricted and artificial two-foci
correlations linking single factors in causality
of disease processes. Hence we need no
longer argue whether a disease is caused by
heredity, constitution, disordered chemistry
or physiology, infection, trauma, or
repressed pathogenic emotions. We are no
longer concerned with either-or single-factor
polarities but currently attempt to map out
the widest possible ranges of conditions,
all of which in some way and at some time,
seem to be implicated in a dynamic chain
of causes and effects.*

Roy Grinker, 1966

*But our recent analysis of twenty-nine types
of leukemia and lymphoma in humans
suggests that the critical step in cancer
may be the break of a fragile site near
an oncogene, without either mutations or
viral involvement. The rearrangements that
result from such breaks may bring the
oncogene on one chromosome under the
influence of another type of gene on another
chromosome, a gene with the power to
activate the oncogene.*

J.J. Yunis and W.R. Hoffman, 1985

5 IN CONCLUSION

Correlations in themselves can never prove causal relationships beyond doubt. The author is fully aware that much more research is required to test the validity of hypotheses based on such associations. Laboratory and clinical studies are essential, as are statistical analyses for smaller administrative units than states, counties for example. In addition, the present study neglected many elements for which data was unavailable. Some of these may be of great significance. Sulphur, for example, because of its known affinity for selenium, should clearly be studied. There is also a need for further detailed examination of the suspected relationships between various leukemias and specific herbicides and pesticides.

CANCER: A MODEL

Despite these limitations, the present study appears to provide sufficient evidence upon which to base speculation about the causes of human cancer. Given the scale of the analysis and difficulties with the data and associated statistical techniques, the model developed here must be viewed as very tentative and subject to future revision.

Bulk and Trace Elements

It is known that every element has a spectrum of possible effects on particular plants or animals. For example, selenium can be toxic in seleniferous areas, have no obvious impact in most regions and be very beneficial to the raising of cattle and sheep elsewhere.[1] This apparent contradiction can be understood only by recognizing that the first instance is one of oversupply, the second of balance, and the latter of deficiency. This type of dose dependency can be represented by a dose-response curve. When various concentrations of an element present in a biological system are plotted against effects on that organism, certain phenomena are commonplace. Firstly, large concentrations are often toxic, injurious or even fatal, while trace concentrations of the same element may be very beneficial and indeed essential. Typically, therefore, too much or too little of any bulk or trace element will be associated with particular illnesses.[2] Fluorine, for example, helps prevent tooth decay and stimulates the development of a bone structure that is less likely to fail with old age. Too little fluorine, therefore, causes damage to bones and teeth. The optimum fluorine concentration in drinking water for the reduction of dental caries is about 1 ppm. Fluorine concentrations of between 4 and 6 ppm, however, greatly reduce osteoporosis, a disease characterized by a reduction of bone mass and collapsed vertebrae. Levels of fluoride in water beyond 8 ppm, on the other hand, result in excessive bone formation in the periosteum and calcification of ligaments that usually do not calcify.[3]

The preceding analysis of global cancer mortality suggests that cancer is also associated with such dose-response curves for most, if not all, known bulk and trace elements. However, it appears that this illness is not related to too much or too little of any particular element. Rather, the causes of cancer appear to be multifactorial, the disease being associated with various carcinogens and with elevated, or depressed, levels of several bulk and trace elements and their antagonists, acting on the body as a system. To illustrate, mortality from esophageal cancer appears to be exacerbated by the presence of certain industrial carcinogens and road de-icing salts. It is also very common in areas that are deficient in calcium and selenium (chiefly soft water regions), especially if diets are sodium and phosphorus enriched. This illness also appears to be more prevalent in the presence of mercury, the selenium antagonist.

In contrast, cancer of the biliary passages and liver appears to be most common when magnesium, calcium, phosphorus, zinc, potassium, sodium and strontium levels are elevated. Each specific cancer, therefore, seems to be associated with numerous dose-response curves, interconnected through a series of synergistic and antagonistic relationships. A particular element may be associated with one type of cancer when at elevated levels, yet at the same time may apparently be linked to a reduction of mortality from another, perhaps depending on the intake of other bulk or trace elements. This situation is further complicated by the numerous synergistic relationships that occur between bulk and trace elements and vitamins; and between certain vitamins and sunlight. Also probably of significance are the antagonistic links between some bulk and trace elements and vitamins and alcohol, coffee, aspirin and air pollution.[4]

The Elderly

Any causative model of cancer must also be able to explain why these diseases are most common amongst the elderly. There may be many reasons for this. It is likely that the impact of some carcinogens is cumulative.

It is also possible that the immune system declines in efficiency with increasing age. Both of these processes might explain why the elderly are prone to so many cancers. It is known, however, that certain elements, such as barium, nickel, arsenic and aluminum, accumulate in tissues as they age. For this reason they are most common in the elderly and are, therefore, known as "age elements".[5] In the preceding analysis of the relationship of the distribution of specific cancers with soil and environmental factors in the United States, elevated levels of these elements were almost invariably found to be associated with increased cancer mortality. This was particularly true of barium, the potassium antagonist. If these statistical relationships are correct, then the aging of tissues and the associated accumulation of the "age elements" within them would inevitably make the elderly more cancer prone.

It has also been established that the skin loses much of its ability to make vitamin D as people grow older, and that the elderly produce this vitamin at only half the efficiency of the young.[6] Older people, therefore, have more trouble utilizing calcium. In addition, many spend disproportionate lengths of time indoors, so avoiding sunlight. Elderly people also often have trouble digesting milk and do not drink it, so living on a diet that is calcium poor, while simultaneously avoiding the chief vitamin D fortified food.[7] Among the diseases known to be the result of calcium deficiency amongst the elderly are osteomalacia, the equivalent of rickets, and osteoporosis, a thinning of the bones, often leading to hip fractures. It appears, therefore, that the diets of many of the elderly are very calcium deficient, a fact that may, in part, also account for their proneness to many cancers.

Bimodal Temporal Distributions

Any causative cancer model should also be able to explain why certain neoplasms, for example those of the testes and bone, have bimodal temporal distributions. Mortality from cancer of the testes, in the United States in both races, for example, falls from birth and then begins rising in the 10 to 14 year age group, peaks in individuals aged between 25 and 29 years, then declines until the 55 to 59 year age group, after which time, death from this disease rises to a second but lower peak in the elderly.[8] It might be hypothesized that, in such relatively unusual cancers, the young are disproportionately exposed to certain cancer promoting substances during their period of maximum growth. One such element may be strontium, which is laid down with calcium in large quantities in newly formed bones and teeth. These two elements generally occur together in nature but, in certain regions, strontium levels may be disproportionately high. Under such circumstances, strontium may compete with calcium within the body, perhaps interfering with normal cellular development.

SIGNIFICANCE OF THE MODEL: SPECULATION

It is unclear, to this author, why elevated, or depressed, bulk and trace element levels appear to be associated with, or prevent, cancer in specific body organs and tissues. It is possible that particular oncogenes may be very dependent upon certain elements to function effectively. Where long term imbalances occur, it is possible that these oncogenes malfunction, or cells become more prone to viruses, or to attack by certain carcinogens.

If specific cancers do, indeed, reflect dietary excesses, or deficiencies, of bulk and trace elements, then a complete reversal of these peaks and troughs may assist cancer patients. To illustrate, breast cancer patients, for example, might be encouraged to take selenium supplements, eat low fat diets and increase their exposure to sunlight. Regardless of whether this approach benefits those already suffering from cancer, the preceding analysis suggests various ways of reducing the incidence of this group of diseases. These include a moratorium on the application of de-icing salts, the use of selenium enriched cattle fodder and a revision of various drinking water standards. Mercury appears to be an even greater hazard than generally believed and requires even more rigorous control. However, since much of it is of natural origin, this will be very difficult to achieve.

REFERENCES

1. KELLER, E.A., *Environmental Geology.* 2nd Edition. Columbus: Charles Merrill, 1979, p. 330.

2. *Ibid.*, pp. 330-331.

3. CARGO, D.N. and MALLORY, B.F., *Man and His Geologic Environment.* Reading, Ma.: Addison-Wesley, 1974.

4. KIRSCHMANN, J.D. and DUNNE, L.J., *Nutrition Almanac.* 2nd Edition. New York: McGraw-Hill, 1984, pp. 93-108.

5. KELLER, *op. cit.*, p. 326.

6. HOLICK, F., cited in The Associated Press, "Extra Sun for Elderly Helps Down to Bones", *Times-Colonist* (Victoria, B.C.), Nov. 5, 1985, p. C4. Discussion of article published in *Journal of Clinical Investigation*, Oct. 1985.

7. *Ibid.*

8. BURBANK, F., *Patterns in Cancer Mortality in the United States: 1950-1967.* National Cancer Institute Monograph 33, United States Department of Health, Education and Welfare, 1977, p. 324.